Handbook of Preventive and Therapeutic Nutrition

James M. Gerber, MS, DC
Western States Chiropractic College
Portland, Oregon

AN ASPEN PUBLICATION®
Aspen Publishers, Inc.
Gaithersburg, Maryland
1993

Library of Congress Cataloging-in-Publication Data

Gerber, James M.
　Handbook of preventive and therapeutic nutrition / James M. Gerber.
　　　　　p.　　cm.
　　　Includes bibliographical references and index.
　　　ISBN 0-8342-0318-9
　　　1. Diet therapy.　　2. Nutrition.　　3. Medicine, Preventive.
　　　I. Title.
　　[DNLM: 1. Diet therapy—handbooks.　2. Nutrition Assessment-
　　　　　　　　　-handbooks.　　WB 39 G362h]
　　　RM216.G39　1992
　　　615.8'54—dc20
　　　DNLM/DLC
　　　for Library of Congress　　　　　　　　　　　　　　　　92-22045
　　　CIP

Copyright © 1993 by Aspen Publishers, Inc.
All rights reserved.

Aspen Publishers, Inc. grants permission for photocopying for limited personal or internal use. This consent does not extend to other kinds of copying, such as copying for general distribution, for advertising or promotional purposes, for creating new collective works, or for resale. For information, address Aspen Publishers, Inc., Permissions Department, 200 Orchard Ridge Drive, Suite 200, Gaithersburg, Maryland 20878.

Aspen Publishers, Inc., is not affiliated with the American
Society of Parenteral and Enteral Nutrition

The authors have made every effort to ensure the accuracy of the information herein, particularly with regard to drug selection and dose. However, appropriate information sources should be consulted, especially for new or unfamiliar drugs or procedures. It is the responsibility of every practitioner to evaluate the appropriateness of a particular opinion in the context of actual clinical situations and with due consideration to new developments. Authors, editors, and the publisher cannot be held responsible for any typographical or other errors found in this book.

Editorial Resources: Lenda Hill
Ruth Bloom

Library of Congress Catalog Card Number: 92-22045
ISBN: 0-8342-0318-9

Printed in the United States of America

1　2　3　4　5

To my wife,
Gretchen Newmark, MA, RD
for her professional advice, patience, and loving support.

Table of Contents

Foreword	xi
Preface	xiii
Acknowledgments	xv

Part I   Clinical Protocols

	1	Anemia	3
	2	Arthritis	8
		Rheumatoid Arthritis	11
		Osteoarthritis	11
		Gout	12
	3	Atherosclerosis	13
	4	Cancer	15
	5	Cardiovascular Disorders	24
		Angina Pectoris	24
		Cardiac Arrhythmias	24
		Congestive Heart Failure	25
		Coronary Thrombosis	25
		Intermittent Claudication	26
		Myocardial Infarction	27
	6	Diabetes Mellitus	28
	7	Food Allergy	35
	8	Food Intolerance	42
	9	Gastrointestinal Diseases	46
		Reflux Esophagitis/Hiatal Hernia	46
		Peptic Ulcer	46
		Irritable Bowel Syndrome	48

	Regional Enteritis (Crohn's Disease)	48
	Ulcerative Colitis	49
10	Geriatric Nutrition	50
11	Gynecologic Disorders	62
	Cervical Dysplasia	62
	Dysmenorrhea	62
	Fibrocystic Breast Disease	63
	Menorrhagia/Metrorrhagia	64
	Menopausal Symptoms	65
	Oral Contraceptive/Estrogen Use	65
	Vaginal Yeast Infections and Chronic Candidiasis	66
12	Hypercholesterolemia and Related Lipid Disorders	69
13	Hypertension	75
14	Hypoglycemia and Related Disorders	81
15	Immunity	85
16	Indigestion	91
	Hypochlorhydria	94
	Pancreatic Insufficiency	95
	Biliary Insufficiency	96
	Colonic Bacterial Flora Disorders	97
17	Kidney Stones	100
18	Migraine Headache	102
19	Muscle Cramps	107
20	Musculoskeletal Trauma	109
21	Obesity	114
22	Osteoporosis	122
23	Pregnancy, Lactation, and Infancy	128
24	Premenstrual Syndrome	141

25	Sports Nutrition	145
26	Weight Loss and Weight Control	155
	Bibliography for Clinical Protocols	161

Part II Clinical Assessment

27	History and Examination	169
	Clinical Approach	169
	Patient History	170
	Physical Tests	172
	Laboratory Tests	176
28	Diet Analysis	177
29	Modified Basic Four Food Guide	180
30	Food Group Exchange System	183
	Bibliography for Clinical Assessment	192

Part III Macronutrients

31	Calories	195
32	Alcohol	202
33	Carbohydrates	205
	Simple Sugars	205
	Complex Carbohydrates (Starches)	208
	Clinical Measurement	209
34	Dietary Fiber	212
35	Lipids and Lipid Factors	217
	Occurrence of Dietary Fats	217
	Dietary Fats and Health	218
	Unnatural Dietary Fats	221
	Cholesterol	222
	Dietary Fat and Cholesterol Score	224
	Plant Sterols	227
	Omega-3 Fatty Acids	227
	Omega-6 Fatty Acids	229

		Choline	230
		Inositol	232
		Carnitine	234
	36	Protein	236
	37	Amino Acids	239
		Lysine	239
		Tryptophan	240
		Phenylalanine/Tyrosine	241
		Sulfur-Containing Amino Acids	243
		Taurine	244
		Arginine/Ornithine	245
		Branched-Chain Amino Acids	246
		Bibliography for Macronutrients	248
Part IV		**Micronutrients**	
	38	Vitamins	253
		Vitamin A—Retinol	253
		Vitamin D—Cholecalciferol	256
		Vitamin E—Tocopherol	259
		Vitamin K—Phylloquinone, Menaquinone	263
		Vitamin B1—Thiamine	264
		Vitamin B2—Riboflavin	267
		Vitamin B3—Niacin, Niacinamide	269
		Vitamin B5—Pantothenic Acid	272
		Vitamin B6—Pyridoxine	274
		Folic Acid	277
		Vitamin B12—Cobalamin	280
		Biotin	282
		Vitamin C	284
		Bioflavonoids	288
	39	Minerals	290
		Boron	290
		Calcium	291
		Chromium	296

	Copper	299
	Fluoride	301
	Germanium	303
	Iodine	305
	Iron	307
	Magnesium	310
	Manganese	313
	Molybdenum	315
	Phosphorus	316
	Potassium	318
	Selenium	321
	Silicon	324
	Sodium and Chloride	325
	Vanadium	329
	Zinc	330
	Bibliography for Micronutrients	334

Appendices

A	Prostaglandins and Related Eicosanoids	339
B	Free Radicals and Lipid Peroxidation	343
C	Carbohydrate Biochemistry and Physiology	346
D	Lipid Biochemistry and Physiology	354
E	Protein Biochemistry and Physiology	359
F	Vitamin Biochemistry and Physiology	362
G	Mineral Biochemistry and Physiology	373
	Bibliography for Appendices A–G	383
H	1989 Recommended Dietary Allowances	384
I	1983 Metropolitan Height and Weight Tables	386

Index **389**

Foreword

Nutrition and nutrient therapies are fundamental parts of a real-world health care program. Since our physical bodies are made up of water, proteins, fats, carbohydrates, minerals, vitamins, and so on, it is only logical to learn thoroughly the uses of these same elements to maintain our bodies, to both prevent and combat disease.

For several generations (one might without too much exaggeration say "several degenerations") the currently dominant form of medical care has minimize, belittled, suppressed and in some cases perverted the science and knowledge of nutrition and nutrient therapeutics in favor of the much higher markup modalities of drugs, surgery, ionizing radiation, and chemotherapy. In doing so, the currently dominant form of medical care has literally been losing touch with the real world: the human body, the "object" of human health care, should logically be repaired first with the elements of which it is made. Only if these means fail should we turn to the more radical means of drugs, surgery, ionizing radiation, and chemotherapy.

This misguided era in health care is ending. Unfortunately, it's not ending because the dominant mode of medical care is demonstrably illogical, dangerous, and less effective than nutritional and other natural therapies. Instead, it's ending (in part) because it's literally threatening to bankrupt us!

More importantly, it's ending because the volume of research in nutritional medicine has grown so large that it can no longer be ignored. Not a week goes by without a media report of research about a vitamin, a mineral, or other nutrients.

Any approach to health care (including prescription drug use, surgery, and nutritional therapies) is susceptible to excesses of enthusiasm, erroneous claims, and occasional fraud. Nutritional therapies have suffered from these problems, as have prescription drugs, surgery, and so on. Despite this, there is an enormous body of well-documented research and clinical application in nutritional therapies.

Dr. James Gerber's *Handbook of Preventive and Therapeutic Nutrition* is based solidly on this mass of well-documented research data. It serves as a valuable primer for the health care professional, but is written and organized to be understood by any concerned non-professional as well. Conservative in approach, it emphasizes well-established research in nutritional therapies, leaving developing therapies for advanced practitioners and students of nutritional therapies.

This Handbook demonstrates that nutritional therapy has indeed "come of age," and can, like any other well-established field, be assembled into a quick reference guide format. Fortunately for all of us, Dr. Gerber has done an extremely competent job.

Over the next twenty years, nutritional therapies (which after all are simply applied human biochemistry) will become the dominant mode of health care. Prescription drugs, surgery, ionizing radiation, and chemotherapy certainly have a place, but that place is much smaller than it presently occupies, and will continue to shrink as research in the real functioning of the human body continues. Look forward to updates of Dr. Gerber's Handbook as our knowledge increases; meanwhile, I'm sure we'll all make good use of this valuable first edition!

Jonathan V. Wright, MD
Tahoma Clinic
Kent, Washington

Preface

Handbook of Preventive and Therapeutic Nutrition is designed as a quick reference guide for the busy health practitioner. It assumes thorough training in the principles of diagnosis as well as good common sense. Essential to the successful use of the information presented herein is a healthy respect for the complexities of human biology and behavior as well as a commitment to the judicious use of the often powerful clinical tools of the science of nutrition.

In Part I clinical protocols are outlined for most of the disorders and conditions in which nutrition may be useful as a primary or adjunct intervention. Part II provides an overview of clinical nutrition assessment along with specific tools for diet analysis and diet prescription. In Parts III and IV the clinical aspects of the various macronutrients and micronutrients are described to increase familiarity with their application in the prevention and treatment of human disease. The appendices provide an outline of nutrition biochemistry and physiology as well as essential reference tables.

As primary health care providers we attempt to help our patients find relief from their ailments and try also to educate them as to how they might prevent future suffering by learning and implementing techniques of health self-enhancement. Thus health practitioners must learn and utilize principles of disease *prevention* as well as therapeutic intervention. In this regard nutrition may play an important, if not vital, role.

Nutrition and diet are not panaceas for all patient complaints and conditions. Yet all too often the role of nutrition in the prevention and treatment of human disease is underappreciated. The lack of a complete authoritative consensus on the validity of certain nutrition therapies is unfortunate and further hinders the utilization of this branch of the health sciences. Consequently, each practitioner must seek to understand the limits as well as the potential of this complex and growing field, as he or she must with any therapeutic tool.

A completely referenced review of all of the issues in clinical nutrition would require several volumes and is beyond the scope of this work. Using the authoritative sources cited in the bibliographies, the author has attempted to glean the leading edge of nutrition science, keeping an open mind toward concepts and applications that have not yet been proved valid to the satisfaction of all. At the same time, a healthy degree of skepticism has emerged in over 10 years of study, teaching, and practice, which, it is hoped, has produced a balanced perspective.

Acknowledgments

I thank the administration, faculty, staff, and students of all the chiropractic colleges with which I have been associated for their inspiration and assistance in this project. Special appreciation is given to Drs. Steve Austin, Judy Ritter, Alan Adams, Robert Boal, and Elizabeth Olsen.

Part I

Clinical Protocols

1. Anemia

GENERAL

Incidence

- Anemia is present in 1% of all males.
- Anemia is present in 10% of elderly males.
- Anemia is present in 10% of all females.
- Anemia is present in 15% of elderly females.

Signs and Symptoms

- fatigue, weakness, drowsiness
- pallor, anorexia, gastric disturbances
- headache, vertigo, tinnitus
- irritability, mental dysfunction
- impaired immune defenses

Initial Laboratory Workup

- complete blood count (CBC)
- hemoglobin (Hgb)
- hematocrit (Hct)
- mean corpuscular volume (MCV)—will indicate microcytic, normocytic, or macrocytic anemia
- mean corpuscular hemoglobin (MCH) and mean corpuscular hemoglobin concentration (MCHC)—will indicate hypochromic, normochromic, hyperchromic anemia

- red blood cell (RBC) distribution width (RDW)
- reticulocyte count

Normocytic normochromic anemias are usually, but not always, non-nutritional.

Common Etiologies and Differential Diagnosis

Decreased RBC Production

- Reticulocyte count is not elevated proportionally to the severity of the anemia.
- Decreased RBC production is caused by **bone marrow disorders** as well as deficiencies of iron, folic acid, and vitamin B12.

Increased RBC Loss or Destruction (Non-Nutritional)

- Reticulocyte count is elevated proportionally to the severity of the anemia.
- Increased RBC loss may be caused by **hemorrhage,** which may be occult; therefore, in the presence of apparently normal nutrition, hemorrhage should be ruled out first.
- Increased RBC loss may be caused by **hemolytic anemias** which, when acute, result in rapid decline of RBC count, elevated serum lactate dehydrogenase (LDH) and bilirubin, and decreased serum haptoglobin. (Chronic cases may respond to vitamin E, 400 to 800 IU/d.)

ATHLETIC ANEMIA (NON-NUTRITIONAL)

Athletic anemia is caused by heavy athletic training, which produces increased plasma volume, hemolysis, or microhemorrhage, or all three. See Chapter 25, "Sports Nutrition."

MICROCYTIC HYPOCHROMIC ANEMIA

Microcytic hypochromic anemia is common in infants and adolescent, pregnant, and premenopausal females. *Rule out non-nutritional anemia.*

Clinical Assessment

Chronic Mild Hemorrhage into Stool or Urine

- Occult blood test of stool or urine is positive.

Menorrhagia

See Chapter 11, "Gynecologic Disorders."

Chronic Disease (Liver, Kidney, Autoimmune, Endocrine, Cancer, etc.)

- MCV is normal or low.
- Serum iron and total iron-binding capacity (TIBC) are low.
- Serum ferritin is normal or elevated.
- Iron supplements are *not* indicated.

Thalassemia Minor

- RDW and reticulocyte count are normal.
- RBC is elevated.
- Hemoglobin electrophoresis is positive.
- Thalassemia minor is common among individuals of African, Southeast Asian, and Mediterranean ancestry.

Sideroblastic Anemia

- Serum iron and ferritin are high.
- Cells in peripheral blood smear are abnormal.
- Anemia may respond to alcohol restriction and vitamin B6, 150 mg/d.

Iron-Deficiency Anemia

- Low **MCV** and high **RDW** are highly sensitive indicators.
- Low serum **ferritin** or **transferrin** saturation verifies iron deficiency.

Treatment (Except As Noted Above)

- Give absorbable iron, 100 mg/d, for 8 to 12 months.
- Give vitamin C, 100 mg/d, with iron supplement.
- Reticulocyte count should rise after 1 week of therapy.
- Hemoglobin should rise within 6 weeks.
- Consider hydrochloric acid supplementation if patient is in a high-risk group. See Chapter 16, "Indigestion."
- See "Iron" in Chapter 39, "Minerals."

MACROCYTIC NORMOCHROMIC ANEMIA

Macrocytic normochromic anemia may be caused by metabolic inhibitor drugs used in treatment of cancer, acquired immunodeficiency syndrome (AIDS) and other infections, and to prevent organ transplant rejection. *Rule out non-nutritional anemia.*

Clinical Protocols 7

Clinical Assessment

- If MCV is borderline, check for hypersegmented **neutrophils.**
- **Serum cobalamin** and **serum** or **erythrocyte folate** are most common tests for differential diagnosis.
- Deoxyuridine suppression test is most accurate means of differentiating between folic acid and vitamin B12 deficiency.
- If cobalamin is low, rule out **pernicious anemia** (a more likely cause of vitamin B12 deficiency than diet inadequacy) with the Schilling test.
- Mild **jaundice** and neurological abnormalities appear in advanced vitamin B12 deficiency.

Treatment

- Give vitamin B12, 150 to 300 µg/d, if indicated.
- In pernicious anemia, consider injectable vitamin B12 and rule out **hypochlorhydria** and **pancreatic insufficiency.** See Chapter 16, "Indigestion."
- Give folic acid, 800 µg/d, if indicated.
- Monitor for hematocrit and reticulocyte count elevation in 1 week.
- Consider malabsorption syndromes and drug effects in resistant and recurrent cases.
- See "Folic Acid" and "Vitamin B12—Cobalamin" in Chapter 38, "Vitamins."

2. Arthritis

GENERAL

Arthritis is an area of great speculation and controversy. Some research evidence is available, but many theories must be judged through the experience of the individual practitioner.

Dietary Therapies

Detoxification

Detoxification is the enhancement of eliminative body functions in order to remove the physiologic stress of accumulated metabolic waste products and environmental irritants. Organs of detoxification/elimination are colon, liver, kidney, skin, and lungs.

Colon.
- Improve digestion to decrease delivery of undigested food to colon.
- Increase dietary fiber to speed transit time.
- Restore normal flora with **acidophilic cultures** if indicated.

Liver.
- Reduce metabolic burden with a diet low in fat, refined sugar, and highly processed foods as well as minimal intake of alcohol, drugs, food additives, and other questionable chemicals.
- Ensure optimal cellular function through adequate intake of all essential vitamins and minerals.
- Consider supplemental **lipotropics** if indicated. See Chapter 16, "Indigestion."

Kidney.
- Reduce filtration burden with a diet low in salt and moderate in protein as well as a minimal intake of drugs, food additives, and other questionable chemicals.
- Maintain low specific gravity by drinking 2 to 3 quarts of plain water per day.

Skin.
- Maintain freely open skin pores with regular washing and mild abrasive rubs.
- Exercise regularly as tolerated to the point of perspiration. Consider steam baths or saunas as tolerated.

Lungs.
- Increase exchange of volatile substances with regular aerobic exercise to tolerance.
- Practice yogic or deep-breathing exercises.

Nightshade-Free Diet

Certain wild plants belonging to the Solanaceae, or **nightshade,** family are known to produce crippling conditions in grazing animals. A professional horticulturalist, Norman Childers, observed that his joint pains subsided when he avoided foods belonging to this family. He proceeded to write articles and a book. He collected hundreds of testimonials from his readers attesting to the value of his diet. No formal research has been conducted to test these claims to date.

The nightshade family includes

- tomatoes
- potatoes (white-fleshed)
- peppers (hot and sweet)
- eggplant
- tobacco

Allergy Elimination

- Water fasts and allergen exclusion diets result in reduction or cessation of symptoms in some patients with **rheumatoid** arthritis.
- Elimination regimen may take 2 or 3 weeks to show effectiveness.
- See Chapter 7, "Food Allergy" for complete protocol.

Prostaglandin Modification (Appendix A)

- Reduced intake of dietary animal fats; increased intake of **polyunsaturates;** and intake of supplemental omega-3 fatty acids, 10 to 15 g/d, may produce some relief in **rheumatoid arthritis** within 3 months.
- Omega-6 fatty acids given as evening primrose oil, 3 to 4 g/d, benefit some patients with rheumatoid arthritis.
- Vitamin E may be helpful. In one pilot study, vitamin E, 600 IU/d, gave relief to more than 50% of subjects with osteoarthritis within 1 week.

Free-Radical Prevention (Appendix B)

- Consider free-radical prevention. Discovery of the degenerative and inflammatory effects of oxygen radicals has led to theoretical suggestions that diet can contribute to pro-oxidant or antioxidant conditions in the joints.
- Reduce pro-oxidant nutrients—excesses of **polyunsaturated fats, iron,** and possibly **copper.**
- Stress antioxidant nutrients (within patient tolerance)—vitamins C and E, beta carotene, selenium, zinc, copper, manganese, and the sulfur-containing amino acids.
- The use of antioxidant enzymes (eg, superoxide dismutase) as oral supplements probably is ineffective because these large molecules do not pass into the circulatory system from the gastrointestinal tract.

RHEUMATOID ARTHRITIS

Many potential deficiencies or imbalances of vitamins and minerals have been suggested by blood studies in patients with rheumatoid arthritis. It is not known whether these contribute to the cause of disease or whether they are part of the systemic effects of the disease. An optimal diet or broad-spectrum supplement, or both, may at least improve overall health in these patients.

Dietary Therapies

- Consider **prostaglandin inhibitors** such as omega-3 fatty acids, omega-6 fatty acids, vitamin E, and bioflavonoids (see above).
- Consider **food allergy** testing.
- Consider calcium supplementation. Calcium pantothenate, 2000 mg/d, produced significant relief in patients with rheumatoid arthritis in one controlled study.

OSTEOARTHRITIS

Dietary Therapies

- **Weight loss,** when indicated, is a primary therapeutic goal in degenerative joint disease. Improvement is seen even in non-weight-bearing joints.
- Consider **vitamin E** and other antioxidants.
- Consider **niacinamide.** Niacinamide, 1000 to 4000 mg/d, according to severity, relieves symptoms and improves joint range of motion, according to one medical researcher who followed hundreds of cases.
- Consider **glucosamine.** Glucosamine sulfate, a breakdown product of chondroitin sulfate, has been successfully used in Europe as an oral treatment for osteoarthritis. Doses begin at 1500 mg/d.

- **dl-Phenylalanine,** 1500 to 2500 mg/d, helps some patients cope with unremitting pain.

GOUT

Dietary Therapies

Purine Restriction

Dietary purine restriction reduces serum uric acid and urinary excretion of urates, although this is not always considered necessary if medication is effective. The following foods should be avoided:

- foods high in purine: **organ meats,** sardines, anchovies, fish roe (eggs)
- foods moderate in purines: animal meats, **seafood,** legumes, spinach

Additional Dietary Measures

- **Weight loss,** if the patient is obese, may relieve symptoms, especially in weight-bearing joints.
- Restrict alcohol, especially beer.
- Increase **fluid** intake and emphasize **alkaline-ash** foods (milk products, most vegetables and fruits) over acid-ash foods (cheese, meat, legumes, grains, cranberries, plums, prunes) to minimize risk of kidney stones.

Supplement Considerations

- Avoid large doses of niacin or retinol.
- High-dose folic acid and vitamin C have positive effects on uric acid metabolism but have not been shown to improve symptoms. Avoid acidic vitamin C because of kidney stone risk.

3. Atherosclerosis

DEFINITION

Atherosclerosis is occlusion of an artery by a process of thickening of the inner wall and accumulation of lipid deposits, fibrous tissue, and cellular debris. It decreases blood flow to distal parts and increases risk of myocardial, cerebral, and renal infarctions.

INITIATING FACTORS

Certain vascular "irritants," many of which depend on dietary or life style factors, may cause the initial lesion that will eventually progress to atherosclerosis.

Atherogenic Factors

- high blood pressure
- cigarette "tar"
- elevated plasma low-density lipoproteins (LDL)
- oxidizing agents such as excess iron or copper, certain environmental toxins, free radicals
- oxidized fats and cholesterol from high-temperature cooking, prolonged storage, or dehydration processes
- homocysteine, which may be produced by a high-protein diet low in vitamin B6 or folic acid
- possibly *trans*-fatty acids
- possibly excess vitamin D

- possibly stress hormones
- possibly severe allergic reactions
- (theory refuted that **homogenized milk** contains atherogenic xanthine oxidase)

ACCELERATING FACTORS

- serum cholesterol above 200 mg/dL (Every 1% reduction in serum cholesterol is associated with a 2% reduction in risk of coronary artery disease.)
- increased platelet aggregation
- excessive circulating insulin
- possibly prostaglandin disturbances
- "type A" behavior (time-pressured, short-tempered, highly stressed)

PROTECTIVE FACTORS

- avoidance of atherogenic factors (see above)
- **antioxidants** (vitamin E, vitamin C, selenium, beta carotene, etc.)
- dietary **monounsaturated** fatty acids (See Chapter 35, "Lipids and Lipid Factors.")
- antithrombotic agents (See "Coronary Thrombosis" in Chapter 5, "Cardiovascular Disorders.")

REGRESSION OF ATHEROSCLEROTIC PLAQUES

- Regression of plaques can be accomplished through intensive programs of dietary control, exercise, and stress management (Pritikin, Ornish).
- Serum cholesterol typically must be lowered below 180 to 200 mg/dL. (See Chapter 12, "Hypercholesterolemia and Related Lipid Disorders.")

4. Cancer

NATURAL HISTORY OF CANCER

Several separate defects must occur to a single cell, accumulating typically over a span of about 25 years, before a malignant cell is produced. Each defect must progress through several stages.

Exposure to Carcinogen

- Exposure usually must be persistent.

Activation of Carcinogen

- Activation is required in some instances.
- **Bile acids** and **nitrites** may be converted by bacteria in gastrointestinal tract.
- Noncarcinogenic chemicals may be converted by **liver enzymes.**

Carcinogen Binding to Deoxyribonucleic Acid (DNA)

- Binding occurs if natural scavengers and other protective proteins are eluded or overcome.

Initiation of Cell Mutation

- Initiation occurs if carcinogen binds to or distorts cancer-related portion of gene.

- Mutation survives if cell divides before natural DNA repair processes occur.

Promotion of Mutated Cell

- Accelerated growth under the influence of certain factors allows increased chance of additional mutations (see below).

Additional Mutations of Mutated Cell Line

- Likelihood of multiple mutations is increased with aging, exposure to promoters, and in tissues with high cell turnover (eg, skin, gastrointestinal tract, endometrium).

Tumorigenesis

- Rapid proliferation of mutated cells occurs.

Malignant Transformation

- Accumulated mutations produce characteristics of invasiveness and **metastasis.**

CARCINOGENS

Foodborne Carcinogens

Fifteen thousand chemicals, added intentionally or inadvertently, are found in the US food supply. Many have not been tested for carcinogenicity. Most appear in very small amounts, but synergistic effects are possible.

- agricultural chemicals—organochlorine pesticides, phenoxyacetic herbicides, **ethylene dibromide** (EDB), some fungicides
- cooking byproducts—charred food hydrocarbons, rancid fats, caramelized sugars
- food additives—saccharin
- microbiological products—**aflatoxins** in moldy grains and legumes
- **nitrosamines**—produced (may be inhibited by vitamin C or E) in stomach from nitrites or nitrates in
  1. meats that are cured, smoked, or otherwise processed (ham, bacon, sausage, luncheon meats)
  2. vegetables grown in fertilized soil

Airborne Carcinogens

- tobacco hydrocarbons
- industrial and auto exhaust pollutants
- construction materials (eg, asbestos)

Waterborne Carcinogens

- industrial pollutants—dioxin, polychlorinated biphenyls (PCBs)
- insecticides—dichlorodiphenyltrichloroethane (DDT)

Ionizing Radiation

- ultraviolet rays
- therapeutic x-ray
- nuclear fallout

Viruses

Free Radicals

- produced by uncontrolled biochemical processes in the body (Appendix B)

Common Chemicals

- benzene

Bile Acid Metabolites

Hormones

- Diethylstilbesterol (DES)

CANCER PROMOTERS

Chemicals

- certain hormones
- bile acid derivatives
- some drugs
- tobacco

Dietary Fat

- high total fat intake
- omega-6 fatty acids
- saturated fatty acids

Dietary Protein

- 20% of total calories or more

Alcohol

Food Additives

- saccharin, cyclamate
- butylated hydroxytoluene (BHT) (controversial)

Irritants

- gallstones
- ulcerative colitis
- oral mucosa irritations
- excessive salt intake

Emotional Stress/Cancer Personality

- loss of crucial relationship
- tension over death of parent
- inability to express hostility, tendency to harbor resentment
- tendency toward self-pity
- difficulty in developing/maintaining meaningful long-term relationships
- poor self-image
- basic sense of rejection by one or both parents

Nutritional Insufficiencies

- protein
- vitamins A, B complex, C, E

- selenium, possibly other trace minerals
- insufficient intake of **cruciferous vegetables** which contain protective substances such as indoles and isothiocyanates
- insufficient intake of carotenoids, bioflavonoids, garlic

CURRENT EVIDENCE FOR CANCER RISK

Bladder Cancer

- low socioeconomic status, **tobacco** use
- exposure to β-napthylamine, **benzidine** (industrial workers)
- history of exposure to excess **saccharin,** nitrates, trichloromethanes in water supply
- diets low in vitamin A, yellow-green vegetables

Breast Cancer

- history of early menarche, late menopause, **obesity,** fibrocystic breast disease, use of high-dose **oral contraceptives** or estrogen
- family history of breast cancer
- diets high in saturated and omega-6 polyunsaturated fat, low in monounsaturated and omega-3 polyunsaturated fat
- diets high in meat, protein, alcohol
- diets low in yellow-green vegetables, fiber, antioxidants, copper

Cervical Cancer

- exposure in utero to **DES**
- history of early onset and multiple-partner sexual activity, smoking during puberty, use of high-dose oral contraceptives or **estrogens**
- diets low in vitamin A/beta carotene, vitamin C, folic acid

Colorectal Cancer

- history of obesity, gallbladder removal, **ulcerative colitis**
- family history of colorectal cancer
- diets high in **cholesterol** and saturated and omega-6 polyunsaturated fat, low in monounsaturated and omega-3 polyunsaturated fat
- diets high in meat, protein, **alcohol,** beer
- diets low in fiber, yellow-green vegetables, cruciferous vegetables, antioxidants, calcium

Endometrial Cancer

- high socioeconomic status, **Caucasoid** race
- history of obesity, use of high-dose estrogens without progesterone, **hypertension,** non-insulin–dependent diabetes
- diets high in saturated and **omega-6 polyunsaturated fat,** low in monounsaturated and omega-3 polyunsaturated fat
- diets low in fiber, yellow-green vegetables, beta carotene

Esophageal Cancer

- history of excessive alcohol use, **smoking**
- diets high in **salt,** smoked/charred meat and fish, nitrates/nitrites, pickled foods, moldy foods, hot foods and beverages
- diets low in fruits, yellow-green vegetables, lentils, animal protein (controversial), vitamins A and C, riboflavin, niacin, calcium, magnesium, zinc, molybdenum

Kidney Cancer

- history of obesity (women), smoking
- diets low in copper

Liver Cancer

- history of **hepatitis B** infection
- history of exposure to **aflatoxins,** safrol, nitrosamines, phenobarbital, vinyl chloride
- diets high in mold-contaminated food, pickled foods, **alcohol**
- diets low in protein, fruits and vegetables, copper

Lung Cancer

- family history of lung cancer
- history of **smoking;** exposure to asbestos, smog, gas fumes, nickel, chromate, gamma-radiation
- diets high in **fat,** cholesterol, alcohol
- diets low in yellow-green vegetables, cruciferous vegetables, beta carotene, vitamin A

Ovarian Cancer

- high socioeconomic status
- diets high in animal fats and coffee, low in vegetable fats
- absence of oral contraceptive use

Pancreatic Cancer

- high socioeconomic status
- tobacco use
- diets high in meat and saturated and omega-6 polyunsaturated fat, low in monounsaturated and omega-3 polyunsaturated fat
- diets low in fruits and vegetables

Prostate Cancer

- older men, African American men
- obesity, exposure to cadmium
- diets high in saturated and omega-6 polyunsaturated fat, low in monounsaturated and omega-3 polyunsaturated fat
- diets low in fiber, yellow-green vegetables, beta carotene, selenium

Skin Cancer

- history of exposure to excess sunlight, petrochemicals, other irritations
- diets low in vitamin A

Stomach Cancer

- diets high in salt, smoked/charred meat and fish, pickled foods, nitrates/nitrites
- diets low in vitamins C and E, copper, fruits, cruciferous vegetables
- history of low gastric hydrochloric acid production

5. Cardiovascular Disorders

ANGINA PECTORIS

Definition

Angina pectoris is episodic chest pain or discomfort caused by reduced blood flow to the heart muscle.

Nutrition Therapies

- Magnesium deficiency may increase likelihood of coronary artery spasm.
- **l-Carnitine,** 750 to 1000 mg twice daily, may reduce symptoms.
- **Coenzyme Q,** 150 mg/d, may reduce attacks and nitroglycerine use.
- **Fish oils,** 3 to 10 g/d, may reduce attacks and nitroglycerine use.
- Beta carotene may reduce progression of arterial disease.
- Vitamin E does not appear to be effective.

CARDIAC ARRHYTHMIAS

Definition

Cardiac arrhythmias occur with disruption of the normal pacemaker or conduction systems that control heart muscle contractions.

Nutrition Therapies

- Treat deficiencies of **magnesium** and **potassium.**
- Avoid caffeine and other stimulants.
- Consider **taurine** therapy (preliminary evidence).

CONGESTIVE HEART FAILURE

Definition

Congestive heart failure results from reduced pumping efficiency of the heart muscle due to any of a variety of pathologies. It causes congestion in the pulmonary or systemic circulation.

Nutrition Therapies

- Treat deficiencies of magnesium and potassium.
- **Coenzyme Q,** 100 to 300 mg/d, may reduce symptoms and improve clinical score.
- **Taurine,** 4 to 6 g/d for 1 month, may reduce symptoms and improve clinical score.

CORONARY THROMBOSIS

Definition

Coronary thrombosis is occlusion of coronary arteries by accumulations of platelets and other blood components.

Preventive Measures

Each of the following measures may reduce platelet adhesion:

- Reduce sugar intake.
- Give vitamin E, 400 to 1200 IU/d.
- Give fish oils, 3 to 10 g/d.
- Treat deficiencies of magnesium and selenium.
- Consider vitamin B6, 50 to 150 mg/d (preliminary evidence).

Either of the following measures may reduce platelet adhesion *and* increase fibrinolytic activity:

- Give vitamin C, 1 to 3 g/d.
- Consider garlic, 18 to 25 mg/d as garlic oil or 100 to 125 mg/kg per day as fresh garlic (one clove = 3 g).

INTERMITTENT CLAUDICATION

Definition

Intermittent claudication is extremity pain on exertion due to progressive atherosclerosis of peripheral vessels.

Nutrition Therapies

- Vitamin E, 300 to 1600 IU/d for at least 3 months, is effective.
- Give vitamin C, 500 mg three times daily.
- Consider **l-carnitine;** 2 g twice daily for 3 weeks increased walking distance 75%.
- Consider **fish oils,** 3 to 10 g/d (preliminary evidence).
- Consider **primrose oil** (containing γ-linolenic acid); 3 g/d for 18 months gave 10% improvement.

MYOCARDIAL INFARCTION

Definition

Myocardial infarction results from sudden reduction of blood flow to the heart due to thrombosis, embolus, or vasospasm.

Preventive Measures

- Prevent coronary thrombosis. See "Coronary Thrombosis."
- Prevent coronary vasospasm. See "Angina Pectoris."
- Prevent myocardial irritability. See "Cardiac Arrhythmias."

6. Diabetes Mellitus

INCIDENCE

- Diabetes affects 5% of the US population.
- Diabetes is the fifth-ranked cause of death from disease.
- Ten percent of diabetics are **insulin-dependent** (type I).
- Ninety percent of diabetics are **non-insulin–dependent** (type II).

TYPE I: INSULIN-DEPENDENT DIABETES

Type I diabetes is also known as juvenile onset diabetes.

Etiology

- Type I diabetes is caused by autoimmune-initiated pancreatic beta cell deficiency, which develops rapidly, usually in persons under age 30 years.
- Genetic factors exist yet interact with nongenetic factors such as advanced maternal age and, possibly, virus exposure.

Clinical Signs

- Classic symptoms include **polyuria,** polydipsia, polyphagia, and **weight loss.**
- Urinary glucose test is positive; the test is useful for screening this rapid-onset form of diabetes.

- **Random plasma glucose** level is over 200 mg/dL, accompanied by rapid onset of symptoms.
- **Ketonuria** is present in uncontrolled diabetes.

Dietary Therapies

- These patients will be self-injecting insulin according to dietary intake and exercise habits.
- Best results occur with regular and consistent eating and exercise schedules. Frequent meals or snacks are usually necessary.
- Carbohydrate, protein, and fat should be distributed as evenly as possible throughout the day.
- Recommended diet composition is identical to that for non-insulin–dependent diabetes (see below).

TYPE II: NON-INSULIN–DEPENDENT DIABETES

Type II diabetes is also known as **adult-onset** diabetes.

Etiology

- Insulin resistance, an acquired insensitivity of cells to insulin, develops slowly. Disease becomes apparent usually after age 40 years.
- Genetic factors are predominant yet interact with other factors:
  1. increasing **age**
  2. development of truncal **obesity**
  3. **sedentary** life style
  4. excessive dietary calories and **alcohol,** but not sugar
  5. possible chromium deficiency

High-Risk Criteria

- family history of type II diabetes
- obesity
- increasing age after 40 years
- Native American, African American, Hispanic ancestry
- history of gestational diabetes or delivery of high-birth-weight (over 9 lb) infant
- unexplained peripheral neuropathy, nephropathy, retinopathy, or premature atherosclerosis

Clinical Signs

- Symptoms are usually absent until the condition is advanced.
- **Fasting plasma glucose** level is above 140 mg/dL on two occasions.
- Two-hour postprandial plasma glucose level is above 200 mg/dL.
- Oral glucose tolerance test is positive: plasma glucose level is above 200 mg/dL at 2-hour draw as well as at one earlier draw (30, 60, or 90 minutes) after ingestion of 75-g glucose load.
- Fasting **insulin** levels are normal or elevated, but insulin responses to carbohydrate intake may be subnormal.
- **Glycohemoglobin** or **serum fructosamine** level is elevated. See Chapter 33, "Carbohydrates."
- Signs of early atherosclerosis, neuropathy, nephropathy, and/or retinopathy may be present.

Dietary Therapies

It may be possible to control type II diabetes with diet alone. Patients taking insulin should be managed with attention to dietary guidelines for type I diabetes as well (see above).

- Weight control: Achieving and maintaining **ideal body weight** will decrease insulin resistance. See Chapter 21, "Obesity," and Chapter 26, "Weight Loss and Weight Control."
- Physical activity: Regular, **aerobic exercise** to tolerance will aid in weight control and may directly decrease insulin resistance. Cardiac stress testing should be done before initiating increases in physical activity. Diabetic medications may need to be reduced when physical activity is greatly increased.
- Diet structure:
    1. high in **complex carbohydrates** (60 to 70% of total calories)
    2. high in fiber (40 to 70 g/d or 25 to 45 g per 1000 kcal), emphasizing foods high in soluble fiber with each meal. See Chapter 34, "Dietary Fiber."
    3. low in fat and sugar
- See Chapter 12, "Hypercholesterolemia and Related Lipid Disorders," and Chapter 30, "Food Group Exchange System."
- Consider restricting high **glycemic index** foods (glucose, maltose, honey, instant potatoes, cornflakes, parsnips) (Appendix C)
- Small amounts of **fructose** and artificial sweeteners may be acceptable.
- Limit protein to recommended dietary allowance (RDA) levels to minimize stress to kidneys.
- Restrict sodium to less than 3 g/d.
- Minimize any other **atherosclerotic** risk factors. See Chapter 3, "Atherosclerosis."

Supplement Considerations

- Consider soluble fiber—oat bran (10 to 20 g/d), guar gum (10 to 20 g/d), xanthan gum (12 g/d), glucomannan (3 to 7 g/d) or psyllium (10 g/d) with all meals.
- Chromium, 200 μg/d, or **brewer's yeast,** 9 g/d, may improve insulin sensitivity and improve serum lipids. Effect may be enhanced with 100 mg of **niacinamide.**

- Prevent deficiencies of vitamin B6, vitamin C, copper, manganese, magnesium, potassium, and zinc.
- Preliminary studies suggest that **carnitine** and **coenzyme Q** may be beneficial.
- Contraindications: Fish oils may elevate LDL and fasting glucose in diabetics. **Niacin** (nicotinic acid) impairs glucose tolerance.

Medical Management

Medication is indicated if plasma glucose cannot be kept below 140 mg/dL fasting and below 180 mg/dL 2 hours postprandial.

IMPAIRED GLUCOSE TOLERANCE

Definition and Prognosis

- Blood sugar levels are abnormal, but not high enough to diagnose diabetes.
- Patients tend to develop atherosclerosis at an increased rate.

Clinical Signs

- Patients may present with symptoms of reactive hypoglycemia. See Chapter 14, "Hypoglycemia and Related Disorders."
- Fasting plasma glucose level is between 115 and 140 mg/dL.
- Two-hour postprandial plasma glucose level is between 140 and 200 mg/dL.
- Glucose-insulin tolerance test: Simultaneous measurements of glucose and insulin levels during oral glucose tolerance test may help establish etiology of glucose intolerance.

Dietary Therapies

- Treat with diabetic diet protocol (see above) and minimize any other existing atherosclerotic risk factors. See Chapter 3, "Atherosclerosis."

Gestational Diabetes

See Chapter 23, "Pregnancy, Lactation, and Infancy."

MANAGING DIABETES COMPLICATIONS

- Primary prevention of these complications requires maintenance of normal blood sugar control.
- Glycohemoglobin levels should be maintained below 8%.
- Research for use of therapeutic supplementation is limited.

Neuropathy

- Consider **vegan** diet (no meat, dairy, eggs), which reduced symptoms within 2 weeks in one study.
- **Neuropathy** is associated with deficiency of pyridoxine, therapeutic doses (150 mg/d) may improve symptoms.
- Consider **inositol,** 1 to 2 g/d, which reduced symptoms and increased some measures of nerve conduction in some, but not all, studies.
- Consider **evening primrose oil,** 4 g/d (containing 320 mg of γ-linolenic acid), which may improve nerve conduction.
- Vitamin B12 injections are advocated by some clinicians.

Nephropathy

- **Low-protein diet** (less than 45 g/day) improves prognosis.
- Maintenance of **normal blood pressure** improves prognosis. See Chapter 13, "Hypertension."

Retinopathy and Cataract

- Diets low in fat, cholesterol, and alcohol and high in **linoleic acid** are associated with a reduced incidence of retinopathy.
- Deficiencies of vitamin B12 and magnesium are associated with retinopathy.
- **Vitamin C** may reduce capillary fragility in the retina.
- **Bioflavonoids** in large doses (1 to 2 g/d) may inhibit cataract formation.

Microangiopathy

- Microangiopathy is associated with vitamin C deficiency, especially if serum cholesterol is elevated.
- Microangiopathy is associated with magnesium and phosphorus deficiency.
- **Vitamin E,** 400 IU/d, may improve microcirculation.

7. Food Allergy

CONDITIONS LINKED WITH FOOD ALLERGY

Many of the associations listed below are controversial.

- hay fever, asthma, sinus conditions
- dermatitis, eczema, frequent itching
- infant colic, diarrhea, frequent digestive upset
- cholecystitis, inflammatory bowel diseases
- recurrent infections
- idiopathic edema or congestion
- arthritis
- recurrent headache, including migraine
- Meniere's disease
- thrombophlebitis, vasculitis
- angina pectoris, cardiac arrhythmias
- mood swings, depression, anxiety, insomnia, behavior disorders
- nocturnal enuresis
- recurrent moniliasis (yeast infection)
- chronic fatigue

Self-administered questionnaires (Exhibit 7-1) may help identify likely candidates for further evaluation.

IMMUNE REACTIONS CAUSING FOOD ALLERGY

Anaphylaxis

- Anaphylaxis is the most accepted mechanism for food allergy.
- The reaction is immunoglobulin E (IgE) antibody-mediated.

Exhibit 7-1 Food Allergy Questionnaire

Have you ever been told you have an allergy to food, drugs, air-borne particles, etc.?	YES	NO
Has any blood relative had an allergy?	YES	NO
Do any foods you eat or do any strong smells make you feel bad?	YES	NO

Circle below any condition or symptom that applies to you **now** or in the **past:**

hay fever   asthma   skin rash   frequent itching
colic   diarrhea   frequent digestive upset
frequent infections or congestion anywhere in body
edema (water retention, swelling)   arthritis   recurrent headache
sinus condition   mood swings   depression   anxiety   insomnia
dark circles or bags under the eyes   chronic fatigue
food cravings (describe)
other unexplained or chronic symptoms (describe)

Indicate below how many times in **three** days you eat foods containing each of the following items:

___wheat ___milk ___egg ___corn ___citrus ___soy

___tomato ___pork ___beef ___nuts ___beans ___seafood

___chicken ___coffee ___yeast ___chocolate

What other foods do you eat at least once every three days? (List them below and state how often you eat them.) _____

_____

_____

- Peak reaction occurs within 30 minutes.
- The reaction is *not* dose-dependent.
- Symptoms usually manifest in skin, gastrointestinal tract, or upper respiratory tract. This type of food allergy may contribute to pediatric conditions such as colic, eczema, and recurrent upper respiratory infection.

Immune Complex Formation

- This reaction is IgG antibody-mediated.
- Peak reaction occurs within 3 to 8 hours.
- The reaction is dose-dependent.
- Symptoms may manifest anywhere.

Cell-Mediated Reaction

- This reaction is T lymphocyte-mediated.
- Peak reaction occurs within 24 to 48 hours.
- The reaction is dose-dependent.
- Symptoms may manifest anywhere.

PREDISPOSING CONDITIONS FOR FOOD ALLERGY

Genetic Predisposition

- Family history may identify patients whose symptoms may be caused by food allergy.

Impaired Immune Response

- results from overactivity of immune surveillance
- results from underactivity of immune modulation
- may be inherited or acquired

Digestion/Absorption Disorder

- may allow absorption of inadequately hydrolyzed food components

- suspect faulty protein digestion as well as increased intestinal permeability due to immaturity, disease, effect of alcohol and some prescription drugs

Monotonous Food Selection

- increases likelihood of repetitive exposure of potential allergens to immune system

LABORATORY TESTS FOR ALLERGY

Note: All positive laboratory tests require confirmation by trial elimination and subsequent food challenge (see below).

Cytotoxic Test

- attempts to assess visually the reaction of leukocytes to food extracts under microscope
- considered unreliable and fraudulent

Antibody Tests

- use **radioallergosorbent** (PRIST/RAST), fluoroallergosorbent (FAST), or enzyme-linked immunosorbent (ELISA) methods to detect levels of circulating IgE or IgG
- can measure total IgE as a screening procedure or can test individual foods for sensitization to IgE or IgG (may be prohibitively expensive)
- considered reliable but do not demonstrate cell-mediated allergy

Sublingual Tests

- attempt to provoke symptoms with sublingual doses of food extracts (reaction expected within minutes)
- controversial, not a medically accepted procedure

ALLERGY ELIMINATION DIETS

- Elimination diets are useful for diagnosis of food allergy as well as for initial attempts at relief.
- Some elimination diets may temporarily exacerbate symptoms up to day 4 or later.
- Elimination is considered successful if symptoms are relieved; may take 4 to 21 days.

Water Fast

- Advantages: Water fast eliminates all possible food allergens.
- Disadvantages: Water fast is difficult to maintain or contraindicated in some patients.

Hypoallergenic Formulas

- Formulas are commercially available as meal-replacement liquids or powders from pharmacies (Flexical, Vivonex) or nutrition suppliers (Ultrabalance, Ultraclear). Protein content must be predigested or amino acid-based. There must be no artificial ingredients.
- Advantages: Formula use attempts to eliminate all possible food allergens, maintains normal nutrient intake.
- Disadvantages: Formulas are expensive and monotonous. Very sensitive patients may not tolerate these formulas.

Hypoallergenic Food Diet

- A hypoallergenic food diet attempts to allow patient to eat fairly normally while eliminating all but most hypoallergenic foods.
- Example: Patient is allowed to eat only lamb, 100% rice products, and pears.
- Advantages: A dietary approach is inexpensive and can approximate normal eating.
- Disadvantages: These diets can be monotonous and may not eliminate all of patient's allergens.

Removal of Suspected Foods Only

- Common allergens are eliminated, including wheat, corn, soy, dairy products, eggs, citrus, tomato, seafood, nuts, pork, beef, chicken, coffee, yeast, and chocolate (see Exhibit 7-1).
- Other foods that occur frequently in patient's diet may also have to be eliminated.
- Advantages: This method is inexpensive and allows more food choices.
- Disadvantages: All of the patient's allergens may not be eliminated.

ALLERGY CHALLENGE TEST

- This test should be done only after successful elimination (symptoms have regressed).
- Food is reintroduced as one food species (eg, milk, egg, cooked wheat) at a time, prepared without additives of any kind (spices, cooking oil, butter, etc.).
- Adequate time after each challenge must be allowed to wait for symptoms to appear before additional challenges are attempted. A 24-hour interval is recommended.

- Foods that do not provoke symptoms may be added to the elimination diet.

ALLERGY TREATMENT

- Foods that provoke symptoms must be eliminated for up to 6 months, at which time another challenge may be attempted. If there is no response, food may be rotated into the diet once every 4 to 7 days.
- Desensitization by intradermal injection (standard allergy treatment) or sublingual ingestion (controversial) may build resistance to some allergens.
- Attention to aspects of prevention may improve response to treatment (see below).

FOOD ALLERGY PREVENTION

Infants

- See Chapter 23, "Pregnancy, Lactation, and Infancy."

Adults

- High-risk individuals should follow a rotation diet, in which all potential allergens are eaten only once every 2 to 4 days.
- Improve digestion, especially of proteins. See Chapter 16, "Indigestion."
- Avoid other predisposing conditions when possible (see above).

8. Food Intolerance

Food intolerance does not involve the immune system; that is, it is not an allergic reaction.

MALDIGESTION DISORDERS

- These disorders are caused by deficiencies of **hydrochloric acid,** pancreatic enzymes, bile acids, **lactase.**
- Symptoms are usually limited to the **gastrointestinal tract.**
- These disorders may require replacement therapy. See Chapter 16, "Indigestion."

GASTROINTESTINAL DISEASE

Celiac Sprue

- Gluten foods (wheat, rye, barley, oats) cause intestinal atrophy and malabsorption.

Cystic Fibrosis

- This disease causes pancreatic insufficiency. See Chapter 16, "Indigestion."

Cholecystitis

- Fatty foods cause severe gallbladder pain.

METABOLIC DEFECTS

Phenylketonuria

- Protein foods, aspartame may cause neurologic reactions, retardation in children.

Galactosemia

- Dairy foods cause vomiting and failure to thrive in infants.

Glucose-6-Phosphate Dehydrogenase Deficiency

- Fava or broad beans produce hemolytic anemia.

PSYCHOLOGIC REACTIONS

- Unpleasant experience associated with certain foods may be relived when the food is eaten again.
- Individuals with vague, transitory complaints may become convinced that certain foods provoke their symptoms, which may cause true psychosomatic reactions to the foods.

NATURAL SUBSTANCES CAUSING FOOD INTOLERANCE

Phenylethylamine

- May cause headaches or other reactions from eating chocolate.

Tyramine

- May cause headache, rashes, or hypertensive reactions from consuming red wine, aged cheese or other fermented foods, brewer's yeast, or canned fish.

Histamine

- Small amounts in fermented foods, sausage, or canned fish, may cause headache, rash or hypotensive reaction.

Histamine-Releasing Agents

- Agents are present in shellfish, chocolate, strawberries, tomatoes, peanuts, pork, wine, and pineapple. Reactions are similar to those to histamine.

FOOD ADDITIVES CAUSING FOOD INTOLERANCE

Tartrazine (Yellow No. 5)

- May cause asthma, rash, or hives from eating yellow, red, or orange-colored processed foods.

Benzoic Acid

- This common preservative in soft drinks and processed foods may cause asthma, rash, or hives.

Sulfites

- May cause anaphylaxis or asthma from consumption of salad, potatoes, and avocado dips in restaurants; dried fruit, wine. Sulfites are banned from salad bars in some states.

Monosodium Glutamate (MSG)

- This widely used flavor enhancer may cause headache and dizziness in susceptible persons, seizures in epileptics.

MICROORGANISM CONTAMINATION CAUSING FOOD INTOLERANCE

Proteus

- Produces a heat-stable toxin in unrefrigerated scombroid fish (tuna, bonita, mackerel) that causes dermatitis and gastrointestinal distress.

Gonyaulax catenella

- This shellfish organism, which causes red tide, produces a heat-stable toxin that causes numbness and paralysis.

9. Gastrointestinal Diseases

REFLUX ESOPHAGITIS/HIATAL HERNIA

Clinical Features

- "heartburn" symptoms
- common in older persons, obese persons

Therapy/Management

- Avoid lying on back after eating and during sleep.
- Avoid compression of abdomen by clothing or posture.
- Normalize body weight.
- Consume small meals only, no food within 4 hours of bedtime.
- Avoid foods that irritate tissue or relax sphincter (Exhibit 9-1).

PEPTIC ULCER

Clinical Features

- pain usually when stomach is empty (duodenal ulcer)
- four times more common in men than women

Therapy/Management

- Bland or Sippy (milk) diet no longer is considered effective.
- Unrefined, high fiber diet may be effective.

Exhibit 9-1 Substances Causing Upper Gastrointestinal Symptoms in Some Patients

Lower esophageal sphincter inhibitors

progesterone
fat
caffeine
chocolate
alcohol
nicotine
peppermint oil
spearmint oil

Gastric secretagogues

methylxanthines (caffeine, theobromine)
decaffeinated coffee
alcohol
cola drinks
tobacco

red pepper
protein and amino acids
niacin
calcium

Mucosal irritants

aspirin
alcohol
caffeine
corticosteroids
bile salts
phenylbutazone (butazolidin)
indomethacin (indocin)
reserpine
black pepper
chili pepper
vinegar
mustard
cloves
nutmeg

- Avoid gastric **secretagogues** and mucosal irritants (see Exhibit 9-1).
- Consume no bedtime snacks.
- Rule out food sensitivities.
- **Zinc,** 100 mg/d, reduced pain and shortened healing time in one study.
- **Glutamine,** 400 mg before meals and at bedtime, shortened healing time in one study.
- There are anecdotal reports of benefit from cabbage juice, 1 qt/d.
- Avoid nicotinic acid supplements.

IRRITABLE BOWEL SYNDROME

Clinical Features

- chronic recurrent abdominal pain with constipation or diarrhea, but no signs of bleeding or inflammation
- most common chronic gastrointestinal disorder
- stress-related

Therapy/Management

- Consider **high-fiber,** low-refined-carbohydrate diet, including supplemental **bran**/psyllium husk as tolerated.
- Avoid gas-forming foods (onion, beans, melon, cabbage, etc.).
- Rule out lactose intolerance.
- Rule out other food sensitivities.
- Stress management techniques are essential.
- Peppermint oil, three to six capsules or 20 drops per day, may relieve symptoms.
- Consider *Lactobacillus acidophilus* therapy.

REGIONAL ENTERITIS (CROHN'S DISEASE)

Clinical Features

- severe cramping and diarrhea
- malabsorption of nutrients
- weight loss

Therapy/Management

- Consider hypoallergenic formula diet during active disease.

- Consider high-protein, high-micronutrient diet, including supplements.
- Avoid sugar and other refined carbohydrates.
- Rule out lactose intolerance.
- Rule out other food sensitivities.
- Monitor serum proteins, complete blood count.
- Consider **glycosaminoglycan** (cartilage extract) therapy.
- **Glutamine** supplementation may provide additional energy source for intestinal tissue.

ULCERATIVE COLITIS

Clinical Features

- episodic cramping and bloody diarrhea
- most common in young adults
- may be accompanied by systemic symptoms
- high risk for future colon cancer

Therapy/Management

- Consider low-residue, lactose-free diet with fluid and electrolyte replacement during exacerbations.
- Consider normal fiber, high-protein (up to double RDA) and micronutrient diet, including supplements.
- Monitor serum proteins, electrolytes, and complete blood count.
- Psyllium husk, oat bran, or pectin may ameliorate diarrhea.
- Avoid sugar and other refined carbohydrates.
- Rule out food sensitivities.
- Consider glycosaminoglycan (cartilage extract) therapy.

10. Geriatric Nutrition

MACRONUTRIENT NEEDS OF THE ELDERLY

Calories

- Calorie requirements decline 20% to 30% with age because of decreasing metabolic rate and reduced physical activity.
- Estimated average RDA for persons over age 51 years is as follows:
  1. men—2300 kcal/d or 30 kcal/kg of body weight
  2. women—1900 kcal/d or 30 kcal/kg of body weight
- Variation among similar individuals may be ±20%. Values will be lower for persons over age 75 years and for those with debilitating disease.
- Lifelong calorie restriction in animals has been shown to increase longevity and reduce age-related morbidity. No human studies have been attempted.
- Nutritional intervention to increase energy intake by 500 kcal/d and to provide at least RDA levels of vitamins and minerals resulted in improved immune response in healthy elderly subjects. A subsequent study incorporating physical fitness training as well as nutrition intervention demonstrated even more dramatic results.

Carbohydrate, Dietary Fiber, and Fat

- Recommended carbohydrate, dietary fiber, and fat intakes are the same as for younger adults. See Chapter 33, "Carbohydrates,"

Chapter 34, "Dietary Fiber," and Chapter 35, "Lipids and Lipid Factors."
- Changing to a high-fiber or restricted fat diet may be impractical or stressful for persons over age 70 years.

Protein

- Protein intake averages 75 to 80 g/d for men, 55 to 65 g/d for women.
- Daily protein intake of 1 g/kg of body weight may be required to maintain protein balance in most healthy elderly persons. This should represent 12% to 14% of total calorie intake.
- Protein is required to prevent accelerated loss of muscle mass.
- Essential amino acids should comprise 30% of total amino acid content.
- Requirement may increase 50% to 100% after physiologic stresses such as surgery, major infection, or trauma.
- High protein intake may be contraindicated in cases of impaired renal function.

Water

- Elderly persons are more prone to dehydration. Their thirst responses may be inadequate and/or renal concentrating ability may be impaired. Requirements also increase with overuse of diuretics and laxatives, chronic diarrhea, vomiting, and hemorrhage.
- Recommended intake is 64 oz (eight cups) of fluid daily.
- Caution: Water intake must be limited in some cases of chronic renal disease and congestive heart failure, and in persons with low serum albumin.

VITAMIN NEEDS OF THE ELDERLY

Vitamin A

- Vitamin A is well absorbed and well conserved in the elderly.
- Chronic excessive supplementation of retinol may not be well tolerated, especially in those with liver or kidney disease.
- **Beta carotene,** 15 to 60 mg/d, may improve immune function in healthy elderly persons.
- High intake of **carotenoids** does not appear to be harmful.

B Complex Vitamins

- Intake varies widely depending on institutionalization, race, socioeconomic status, health status, medications, and alcohol use. See Chapter 32, "Alcohol."
- Dietary inadequacies or low biochemical indicators are found in a greater proportion of elderly persons for many B vitamins, especially vitamin B6, and **folic acid.**
- Up to 20% of elderly persons may develop irreversible impairment in vitamin B6 utilization.
- Up to 40% of older elderly persons have atrophic gastritis that impairs vitamin B12 and folic acid bioavailability.
- Deficiency of folic acid due to poor absorption is improved in elderly patients with atrophic gastritis by supplementing hydrochloric acid.
- Caution: Niacin supplements taken with vasodilating hypertension medications may cause postural hypotension.
- Caution: Vitamin B6 supplements reduce the effectiveness of L-dopa in Parkinson's disease.

Vitamin C

- Antioxidant effect may delay many types of age-related pathologies.
- Dietary intake as well as serum levels are inadequate in many elderly persons, especially those who are institutionalized.

Vitamin D

- Many changes in life style or physiologic function may predispose the elderly to low vitamin D status. See "Vitamin D—Cholecalciferol" in Chapter 38, "Vitamins."
- Many elderly persons have reduced levels of serum 25-hydroxyvitamin D_3 and/or serum 1,25-dihydroxyvitamin D_3.
- Supplementation of 400 IU/d has been suggested as a prudent preventive strategy if serum calcium is monitored.
- Caution: Excessive doses taken with digitalis may precipitate cardiac arrhythmias.

Vitamin E

- Antioxidant effect may delay many types of age-related pathologies.
- A dose of 800 IU/d has improved **immune response** in healthy elderly persons.
- Caution: Vitamin E taken with anticoagulant medication may increase risk of hemorrhage.

Vitamin K

- Over 50% of elderly persons may have impaired vitamin K status.
- Vitamin K may play an important role in **osteoporosis** prevention.

MINERAL NEEDS OF THE ELDERLY

Calcium

- Up to 1500 mg/d is necessary to preserve calcium balance in many elderly persons. Negative calcium balance will aggravate age-related bone loss. See Chapter 22, "Osteoporosis."
- Caution: Supplements taken with calcium channel blockers may aggravate pre-existing cardiac arrhythmia.

Chromium

- Deficiency probably occurs in many elderly persons, especially those consuming diets high in refined carbohydrates.
- Supplemental chromium has improved **glucose tolerance** and serum lipid levels in some elderly subjects.

Copper

- Deficiency probably occurs in many elderly, especially if rich dietary sources (liver, shellfish, nuts, legumes, whole grains) are not regularly consumed or if high-dose vitamin C or zinc supplements are used.
- Copper deficiency may play a role in the pathophysiology of many age-related diseases. See "Copper" in Chapter 39, "Minerals."

Iron

- Iron requirement in postmenopausal women is reduced due to cessation of menses.

- Deficiency is common only in those with conditions causing chronic hemorrhage or those taking large amounts of aspirin or arthritis drugs.
- Deficiency is more likely with excessive tea drinking, low meat intake, and low vitamin C intake.
- Caution: Elderly patients with inflammatory and other chronic diseases may exhibit false signs of iron deficiency. See "Iron" in Chapter 39, "Minerals."

Magnesium

- Deficiency is common in those with gastrointestinal diseases causing malabsorption.
- Depletion is common with chronic use of digitalis and diuretics.

Manganese

- Manganese intake is below recommended levels in some elderly persons.
- Deficiency is more likely in individuals with high-fiber diets and who supplement with calcium or iron.

Phosphate

- Depletion is common with overuse of aluminum or magnesium antacids.

Potassium

- Dietary deficiency is common among those who avoid fruits and vegetables.

- Depletion is common due to overuse of laxatives and diuretics.
- Elderly patients taking supplemental potassium should be monitored for hyperkalemia, especially if kidney dysfunction is suspected.

Selenium

- Only a minority of elderly persons appear to have low intakes of selenium.
- Large doses with vitamin E improved mental status and reduced fatigue and anorexia in one contolled study using elderly subjects.

Zinc

- Deficiency is common in the elderly, especially those with low animal protein diets and high intake of bran products.
- Deficiency is common in those with muscle-wasting diseases, malabsorption syndromes or postsurgical weight loss.
- Depletion is common with chronic use of digitalis and diuretics.
- A dose of 100 mg/d improved immune function in a group of healthy elderly persons.
- Caution: Supplemental zinc should not be given without assurance that copper status will be adequately maintained.

HEALTH CONDITIONS AFFECTING GERIATRIC NUTRITION

Factors Affecting Food Intake

- oral/dental problems
- decreased smell and taste sensations
- vision and motor problems

Clinical Protocols 57

Digestive Impairments

- Reduced gastric secretion impairs protein, vitamin B12, folic acid, and mineral nutrition.
- Reduced absorption increases incidence of **flatulence.**
- Reduced exercise and muscle tone and lower intake of fiber and fluids contribute to constipation and **diverticulitis.**
- Increased incidence of bacterial overgrowth syndromes cause malabsorption of **fat,** protein, carbohydrate, electrolytes, and vitamin B12.

Effects of Hospital Stays

- Adequate food usually is provided but often is not eaten.
- Fifty percent of hospitalized elderly persons have protein-calorie malnutrition.
- Average nutrient intake is below 50% of RDA for vitamin D, vitamin B6, folic acid, zinc, and magnesium.
- Average nutrient intake is between 50% and 70% of RDA for calories, protein, vitamin B3, vitamin B12, calcium, and iron.

DRUG-NUTRIENT INTERACTIONS

Use of the following medications may impair the availability and/or function of the indicated nutrients.

Antiarthritic Drugs

- aspirin—iron, folic acid, and vitamins C, B1, and K
- nonsteroidal anti-inflammatory drugs (ibuprofen, indomethacin, etc.)—iron

- corticosteroids—zinc, calcium, potassium
- colchicine—protein, vitamin A, vitamin B12, potassium
- penicillamine—vitamin B6, iron, copper, zinc

Gastrointestinal Remedies

- antacids—many minerals and vitamins
- mineral oil—fat-soluble vitamins
- chemical laxatives—vitamin D, calcium, potassium
- histamine blockers—vitamin D, vitamin B12
- sulfasalazine—folic acid, iron

Antihypertensives

- diuretics, potassium-wasting—many minerals
- triamterene—folic acid
- hydralazine—vitamin B6

Antihyperlipidemic Medications

- cholestyramine resin, clofibrate, colestipol—fat-soluble vitamins, vitamin B12, many minerals

Cardiac Medications

- digitalis, digoxin—magnesium, potassium, zinc

Psychoactive Medications

- barbiturates—vitamin D, folic acid
- phenytoin (Dilantin)—vitamins D and K, folic acid
- primidone—vitamins C, D, K, and B12, folic acid

Antibiotics

- isoniazid—vitamins D, and B6, folic acid
- tetracycline—calcium, vitamins C, K, B2
- cephalosporin—vitamin K
- rifampin—vitamins D, B3, B6

SENILE DEMENTIA

Occurrence

- mild in up to 15% of over-65 population
- severe in up to 6% of over-65 population
- prevalence of 20% to 36% in over-85 population
- 10% to 20% considered treatable

Nutritional Deficiencies/Excesses

- Five percent of total cases are related to deficiencies in vitamin B1, B3, B12 or folic acid.
- Dementia can be caused by excesses of alcohol (10% of elderly), aluminum (dialysis), and manganese (occupational).

Stroke

- Of total dementia cases, 5% to 15% are related to multiple infarcts (stroke), which are preventable by controlling alcohol intake, hypertension, diabetes, and hypercholesterolemia.
- Risk increases with
    1. increasing age
    2. male gender (until 75 years)

3. family history
4. African American race
5. elevated systolic blood pressure (2 to 4 times higher risk)
6. previous strokes (20% chance of recurrence)
7. history of heart disease or surgery
8. diabetes (2 times higher risk)
9. oral contraceptive use
10. smoking
11. increased blood viscosity
12. alcohol and drug abuse

ALZHEIMER TYPE

- 50% to 60% of dementia cases
- 11% of over-85 population
- genetic factor exists
- not considered nutrition-related
- development of memory problems, followed by social and vocational difficulties, inability to handle routine tasks, disorientation in familiar surroundings
- progressive intellectual impairment and deterioration of motor skills, often eventual incontinence and confinement to bed
- predisposes victims to nutritional deficiencies because of abnormal eating behaviors or feeding difficulties

Nutritional Considerations

- Agitated or institutionalized victims may lose weight continuously unless they receive supplements with sufficient calories.
- Fortified beverages and puddings can meet 25% to 70% of nutritional needs.
- Consider avoidance of aluminum pots, utensils, and medications (many antacids, buffered analgesics, and other gastrointestinal

remedies), as reduced capacity to eliminate this metal may exist in some elderly.
- In early cases, consider choline, 10 g/d, or high-potency lecithin (phosphatidylcholine), 30 g/d.

PARKINSON'S DISEASE

Nutritional Considerations

- Avoid taking medications with high-protein meals, which reduce absorption of L-dopa.
- Avoid wheat germ or vitamin B6 supplements, which increase breakdown of L-dopa.
- Avoid choline or tryptophan supplements, which antagonize dopamine production.
- Do not restrict salt if hypotension is a side effect.

11. Gynecologic Disorders

CERVICAL DYSPLASIA

Definition

Cervical dysplasia is the presence of precancerous cell changes indicated by an abnormal Papanicolaou (Pap) smear (class III).

Nutrition Therapies

- **Folic acid,** 10 mg/d, has resulted in 1 classification point improvement in abnormal Pap smears.
- **Vitamin A** deficiency may be involved or retinol metabolism may be deranged. Some practitioners give megadoses of 50,000 to 60,000 IU/d on a short-term basis.
- Increased **nutritional antioxidants** (beta carotene, vitamins C and E, selenium) are advisable.

DYSMENORRHEA

Definition

Dysmenorrhea is painful menstruation.

Pathophysiology

- Rapid drop in progesterone level stimulates excess production of 2-series prostaglandins, which

1. increases myometrial irritability
  2. reduces local blood flow causing ischemia and congestion
  3. increases peripheral nerve sensitivity.
- Rule out pelvic abnormalities.

Nutrition Therapies

- Vitamin E, 200 IU/d, during the second half of menstrual cycle was effective in 68% of subjects compared with 18% of controls.
- Magnesium and vitamin B6, 400 mg/d each throughout the cycle, and 100 mg each every 2 hours as needed during menses, decreased intensity and durations of cramps over 4 to 6 months in subjects with reduced RBC magnesium levels.
- **Niacin,** 200 mg/d for 7 to 10 days premenstrually, and 100 mg every 2 to 3 hours as needed during menses, helped about 90% of 80 subjects over a 3-year follow-up. **Vitamin C** and **bioflavonoids** may enhance effectiveness.
- Calcium, 1000 mg/d, reduced symptoms in 33 subjects.
- Prostaglandin mechanism of this disorder suggests that essential fatty acids (linseed or safflower oil, 1 Tbs/d; γ-linolenic acid, 240 mg/d; or fish oils, 5 g/d) may be effective (clinical studies are not available).
- See also Appendix A.

FIBROCYSTIC BREAST DISEASE

Definition

Fibrocystic breast disease is characterized by painful cystic lesions in the breast, which are worse premenstrually.

Nutrition Therapies

- Methyl xanthine restriction (avoidance of caffeine and related chemicals found in tea and chocolate) reduced signs and symptoms in some, but not all, subjects; 100% compliance improves outcome.
- **Vitamin E,** 200 to 600 IU/d, reduced signs and symptoms in some, but not all, studies.
- **Evening primrose oil,** 3 g/d (containing 240 mg of γ-linolenic acid) demonstrated subjective and objective improvement in two studies.
- The effectiveness of **choline,** 500 mg/d, with inositol, 500 mg/d, has been reported.
- Animal studies suggest that iodine deficiency worsens the effect of estrogen on cystic lesions.
- Rule out thyroid dysfunction.

MENORRHAGIA/METRORRHAGIA

Definitions

Menorrhagia is excessive bleeding during the menstrual period; metrorrhagia is bleeding between menstrual periods.

Nutrition Therapies

- Iron deficiency anemia is common and may worsen the condition. Consider iron supplementation, up to 100 mg/d, especially if serum ferritin is low.
- Vitamin A, 25,000 IU twice daily for 15 days, resulted in 57% complete relief and 35% some improvement among 71 subjects.
- Bioflavonoids and vitamin C, 600 mg/d each, reduced symptoms in 14 of 16 subjects.

- Consider prostaglandin imbalances (Appendix A).
- Rule out pelvic abnormalities and thyroid dysfunction.

MENOPAUSAL SYMPTOMS

Definition

Menopausal symptoms include vasomotor instability ("hot flashes"), vaginal atrophy, and depression.

Nutrition Therapies

- **Vitamin E,** 300 IU/d or less, improved vasomotor and other symptoms in most subjects in several older studies.
- **Bioflavonoids,** 500 to 3000 mg/d, were reported to control vasomotor flushing in one study.
- Ginseng therapy was reported to be effective in one case of vaginal atrophy. It is contraindicated in hypertension.

ORAL CONTRACEPTIVE/ESTROGEN USE

- decreases absorption of water-soluble vitamins, especially vitamin B6 and folic acid
- alters glucose tolerance and increases serum glucose and triglycerides
- reduces calcium loss from bone

PREMENSTRUAL SYNDROME

See Chapter 24, "Premenstrual Syndrome."

VAGINAL YEAST INFECTIONS AND CHRONIC CANDIDIASIS

Vaginal Candidiasis

- Fastidious hygiene must be observed.
- Avoid antibiotics when possible, especially tetracycline, which may destroy normal protective flora and promote growth of yeasts.
- Boric acid suppositories, 600 mg at bedtime for 14 nights, is reported to be effective.
- High-dose ascorbic acid may increase acidity of vaginal secretions.
- Acidophilic douches are reported to be effective. Use plain yogurt with addition of 10 to 12 capsules of acidophilic culture or equivalent at bedtime; use a vinegar douche next morning (1 Tbs of vinegar per quart of water).
- Consumption of one cup of yogurt per day or four to six capsules of acidophilic culture per day is reported to reduce frequency of vaginal yeast infections.
- Rule out zinc deficiency.
- Rule out glucose intolerance with resulting increase in glucose content of vaginal secretions.

Systemic Candidiasis

Systemic candidiasis is a controversial diagnosis except in cases of severely immunocompromised patients. No adequate research exists for the following indications and treatments.

Benchmarks in Patient History

- chronic vaginitis
- broad-spectrum antibiotic therapy, corticosteroid therapy

- chronic allergies
- defective cellular immunity, immunosuppressant therapy
- oral contraceptive use, recent pregnancy

Additional Symptoms

- itching
- gastrointestinal distress
- psychologic manifestations
- reproductive organ disorders
- skin problems

Clinical Assessment

- To date, there is no reliable test to prove the existence of this infection except in severely immunocompromised patients.
- Rule out immunosuppression disorders (AIDS, etc.), hepatitis.

Dietary Therapies

- Avoid alcohol, sugar, juice, and sweet or dried fruits.
- Consume other fruits sparingly.
- Avoid cheese and other milk products if they cause distress.
- Avoid fermented foods (sourdough bread, pickles, vinegar).
- Avoid everything containing or derived from any yeast.
- Avoid mushrooms or other fungi.

Supplement Considerations

- high-potency lactobacillus culture
- digestive enzymes and hydrochloric acid
- garlic
- essential fatty acids (γ-linolenic acid or fish oils) with vitamin E
- basic mineral support

- no B vitamins if sensitive
- caprylic acid
- oleic acid (olive or canola oil)
- biotin

Medications

- oral antifungal agents (nystatin, etc.)

12. Hypercholesterolemia and Related Lipid Disorders

INCIDENCE

At least 25% of the adult US population has serum cholesterol levels over 200 mg/dL.

EVALUATION

- National Institutes of Health criteria are used here.
- Some references use millimole units instead of milligrams per deciliter. One millimole = approximately 39 mg/dL.
- Ideal serum cholesterol values are below 200 mg/dL.
- Values above 240 mg/dL require verification and further analysis in all cases.
- Values from 200 to 240 mg/dL require verification and further analysis in younger patients or if additional coronary risk factors exist, such as
  1. male gender
  2. cigarette smoking (more than 10 per day)
  3. hypertension
  4. severe obesity (30% or more above ideal)
  5. diabetes
  6. family history of premature (before age 55) coronary heart disease
  7. diagnosed cerebrovascular or peripheral vascular disease
  8. low high-density lipoprotein (HDL) cholesterol (below 35 mg/dL)

- If two major risk factors exist *or* the individual already has a history of atherosclerotic heart disease, LDL cholesterol should be measured. LDL values above 130 mg/dL require intervention in these high-risk cases. LDL values above 160 mg/dL require intervention in all cases.
- Many laboratories report the ratio of total cholesterol/HDL or LDL/HDL along with statistics that predict coronary disease risk. Above-average risk levels require intervention.
- Children and adolescents from families with hypercholesterolemia or premature cardiovascular disease should maintain serum cholesterol levels below 170 mg/dL *or* serum LDL levels below 110 mg/dL. Elevated levels should be addressed as in adults.
- Contributing disorders (thyroid, kidney, liver disease, diabetes) and drug effects must be ruled out.
- Patients with extreme elevations (total cholesterol over 300 mg/dL) should be evaluated for genetic hyperlipidemias.
- New research indicates that apoprotein ratios are excellent predictors of coronary disease risk. Apoproteins reside on specific lipoproteins and influence cholesterol metabolism (Appendix D).

THERAPEUTIC OVERVIEW

- Reduce dietary saturated fat and cholesterol as much as possible. No dietary need exists for these substances.
- Maintain total dietary fat below 30% of total calories, emphasizing monounsaturated and some polyunsaturated fats.
- Restrict sugar intake in glucose-intolerant patients.
- Increase dietary **fiber,** especially soluble fiber.
- Restrict alcohol to two drinks or less per day.
- Control **weight** to within 10% of ideal body weight.
- Advise aerobic **exercise** (minimum 30 minutes at 60% of maximal heart rate three times per week) within patient tolerance.

- Treat suspected nutritional deficiencies.
- Consider therapeutic food supplements.
- Consider referral for medication in extreme or resistant cases.

INTERVENTION STRATEGIES

Dietary Fats

Inspect diet for saturated fat/cholesterol sources and help patient make alternative low fat or polyunsaturated fat choices.
- Common offenders include organ meats, red meats, high-fat dairy products, fried foods and snacks, fast foods, eggs, rich pastries and desserts, butter, many sauces and gravies, coffee creamer
- Alternative foods include the following:
  1. breakfast: whole-grain cereals, breads, fruit, low- or nonfat dairy products, egg substitutes
  2. meats: skinless poultry, seafood (not deep-fried), very lean red meats
  3. dairy: nonfat or 1% milk, buttermilk; low-fat cottage, ricotta, or farmer's cheese; part-skim cheeses in moderation; very low or nonfat frozen yogurt
  4. entrees: pasta with meatless sauce, vegetarian bean or pea soups, brown rice and vegetable casseroles, tofu or soybean products, low-fat salad bars
  5. snacks: fruit, vegetables, juices, crackers, pretzels, bagels, air-popped corn, nonfat yogurt, low-calorie desserts
  6. miscellaneous: soft or liquid margarines in moderation, monounsaturated oils (olive, canola, almond, peanut), eggless mayonnaise, low-calorie or no-oil salad dressings
     (a) Caution: Hydrogenated vegetable oil-containing substitutes (hard margarine, shortening) appear no safer than saturated animal fats.
     (b) Caution: Excessive use of polyunsaturated fats as substitutes may increase risk of gallstones and possibly cancer.

- Restaurant dining:
  1. Avoid meat and cheese dishes, sauces, fried foods, rich desserts.
  2. Look for entrees in compliance with American Heart Association (AHA) guidelines, specified in some restaurants.
  3. Seafood, salad entrees, and some ethnic cuisines (Asian, Middle Eastern) may be the best choices.

Dietary Fiber

- Help the patient find food choices high in soluble fiber.
  1. oats, oatmeal and oat bran
  2. whole fruits such as apples
  3. legumes (beans, peas, peanuts)
- Consider supplemental psyllium husk (10 g/d), pectin (6 to 50 g/d), or guar gum (5 to 30 g/d) with meals.

Nutrient Deficiencies

Evaluate and/or treat for possible nutritional deficiencies related to hypercholesterolemia:

- vitamin C, even if only marginally low
- chromium (difficult to assess)
- copper, especially with high zinc intake

Other Dietary Issues

- Olive oil reduces LDL and heart disease risk.
- Soybeans reduce LDL and triglycerides.
- Boiled or percolated coffee increases cholesterol.

Clinical Protocols 73

Therapeutic Supplements

- Consider **fish oils** only if triglycerides are also elevated.
  1. 5 to 10 g/d or 20 to 40 mL/d marine lipid concentrate (eg, proprietary product MaxEPA)
  2. 1.8 g/d pure EPA
  3. oils high in docosahexaenoic acid (DHA) and low in EPA (Check product labels; may be best for reducing LDL while maintaining HDL levels.)
- Consider **niacin,** which lowers LDL and triglycerides and raises HDL.
  1. Begin with 100 mg three times daily with meals.
  2. Increase by 300 mg/d each week up to a maximum of 3 to 6 g/d.
  3. Monitor liver enzymes, uric acid, glucose.
  4. Possible side effects include flushing, headaches, gastrointestinal upset, aggravation of peptic ulcers or gouty arthritis, and cardiac arrhythmias.
- Consider **calcium;** 2 g/d with meals may help bind fats in the gastrointestinal tract.
- Consider **garlic,** 9 g/d fresh (three cloves), 600 mg/d powder, or 18 to 25 mg/d oil.
- Do not recommend lecithin. Recent studies show that effects are solely from polyunsaturated fat content, not phospholipids.

HYPERTRIGLYCERIDEMIA

- If triglyceride level exceeds 250 mg/dL, emphasize
  1. weight normalization
  2. alcohol restriction (zero to two drinks allowed per week)
  3. aerobic physical activity
  4. simple sugar restriction
  5. increased use of fish and fish oils
- Consider niacin therapy if cholesterol is also elevated.

HIGH-DENSITY LIPOPROTEIN DEFICIENCY

- If HDL cholesterol is below 35 mg/dL emphasize
    1. cessation of smoking and heavy coffee drinking
    2. weight normalization
    3. aerobic physical activity
    4. avoidance of anabolic steroids, progesterone-like agents and β-blockers
    5. moderate alcohol intake
    6. avoidance of sugar (may raise HDL in some persons)
- Chromium, 200 μg/d, has been effective.
- Garlic oil, 18 mg/d from 9 g of fresh garlic (approximately three cloves), has been effective.

MONITOR LIPID LEVELS MONTHLY

- After 3 months, consider referral to a registered dietitian in cases of poor dietary compliance.
- After 6 months, consider referral for medication in high-risk cases with poor responses to conservative treatment.

13. Hypertension

INCIDENCE

More than 15% of the adult US population (30% of African Americans) have blood pressure levels over 160/95 mm Hg.

EVALUATION

- National Institutes of Health criteria are used here.
- Diastolic blood pressures over 90 mm Hg and systolic pressures over 140 mm Hg should be reduced.
- Elevated diastolic blood pressures below 105 mm Hg and systolic pressures below 160 mm Hg may be managed without medication for 3 to 6 months.
- Contributing disorders (kidney, endocrine, cardiovascular) and drug effects must be ruled out.
- Target organ damage (cardiovascular, cerebrovascular, kidney) should be assessed.
- Additional cardiovascular risk factors should be identified.

NUTRITION THERAPIES

Weight Reduction

- Weight reduction is usually effective but hard to maintain.
- There is an average rise of 6.5 mm Hg systolic blood pressure for every 10% increase in body weight over ideal weight, especially if increase is in body fat content.

- Weight loss usually requires a combination of lowered calorie intake (less fat and sugar) plus more calorie expenditure (exercise). See Chapter 21, "Obesity," and Chapter 26, "Weight Loss and Weight Control."

Alcohol Restriction

- Allow no more than two drinks per day.
- Alcohol restriction reduces blood pressure and risk of stroke in heavy drinkers.

Sodium Restriction

- Sodium restriction may help 20% to 50% of hypertensives.
- Restrictive diets are useful in patients with normal or low renin levels as measured by plasma renin activity test.
- Sodium restriction is more effective in obese patients.

Mild Sodium Restriction (2500 to 4500 mg/d)

- Mild sodium restriction is adequate for drug-controlled mild hypertension only.
- Mild sodium restriction may enhance herbal diuretic therapy for hypertension.
- No salty foods, table salt, or salty seasonings are allowed. Minimal salt is allowed in cooking. See "Sodium" in Chapter 39, "Minerals."

Moderate Sodium Restriction (1500 to 2500 mg/d, 70 to 100 mEq, 4 to 6 g of Salt)

- Moderate sodium restriction produces better results than mild sodium restriction.

- No salt at all may be used in cooking or eating.
- Most processed foods must be avoided.
- Diet counseling makes compliance more likely.

Dietary Fat Modification

- Lower total fat and saturated fat may reduce viscosity of blood.
- Increasing polyunsaturated fats (vegetable oils, fish oils, etc.) may affect vascular and renal prostaglandins.
- Pritikin diet with exercise may reduce blood pressure by 21/11 mm Hg in nonmedicated patients and by 7/5 mm Hg in medicated patients.
- Fatty fish and fish oils in large amounts may reduce blood pressure up to 15/7 mm Hg.

Potassium Therapy

- Higher potassium intake may vasodilate or assist sodium and water excretion.
- Intake of 5000 to 7000 mg/d (vs. 2000 to 4000 mg/d RDA) produces 3% to 10% drop in blood pressure. Better results are seen in African Americans.
  1. Indications: Patients taking certain diuretics called thiazides or loop diuretics *require* increased potassium intake.
  2. Contraindications: Patients with kidney disease and patients using potassium-sparing diuretics (spironolactone or triampterene family) or angiotensin-converting enzyme inhibitors should *not* increase potassium intake.

Calcium Therapy

- Higher calcium intake may help relax vascular smooth muscle and increase sodium excretion.

- Calcium, 1000 to 2000 mg/d for at least 2 months, may reduce diastolic pressure by 4 to 9 mm Hg and systolic pressure by 6 to 13 mm Hg.
- Best results are seen in those with low serum renin, low/normal serum ionized calcium, and high urinary sodium excretion.

Magnesium Therapy

- Magnesium deficiency can contribute to hypertension. Many diuretics deplete magnesium as well as potassium.
- Magnesium, 360 mg/d for 6 months, reduces blood pressure 12/8 mm Hg in depleted patients.

Caffeine Restriction

- There is no lasting effect in persons accustomed to caffeine.

Exercise Therapy

- Exercise may have temporary acute effect on blood pressure as well as contribute to weight loss and stress reduction.
- Five sets of 10-minute exercise bouts with 3 minutes of rest in between reduces blood pressure 25% for 4 to 10 hours.
- Regular aerobic exercise and moderate-circuit weight-training for 10 weeks reduced blood pressure 14/15 mm Hg.

Stress Reduction

- Identify and minimize sources of stress; explore relaxation therapies and biofeedback.

- Stress reduction, biofeedback, and meditation have been shown to be effective in some, not all, studies.

Heavy Metal Detoxification

- Cadmium and lead accumulation may contribute to hypertension.
- Hair analysis may be useful for screening.
- Vitamin C and nutrient minerals may help lower body burden of toxic metals.

Other Therapeutic Agents

- Consider 6 g/d taurine (preliminary evidence).
- Limited research suggests that coenzyme Q, 100 mg/d, is effective in subjects judged deficient.

DRUG/NUTRIENT INTERACTIONS

Diuretics

- Thiazide (eg, Diuril), furosemide (eg, Lasix) and other potassium-wasting diuretics
  1. cause sodium excretion
  2. cause potassium, magnesium, and sometimes calcium loss
- Spironolactone (eg, Aldolactone) and other potassium-sparing diuretics
  1. cause sodium excretion and potassium conservation
  2. require limitation of dietary potassium

Nondiuretics

- Sympathetic blocking agents (eg, propranolol, methyldopa), vasodilators (hydralazine), and calcium antagonists (nifedipine, verapamil) have no nutritional consequences.

14. Hypoglycemia and Related Disorders

HYPOGLYCEMIA CRITERIA

- Plasma glucose levels are below 50 mg/dL (some say below 60 mg/dL).
- Symptoms are coincident with low plasma glucose.
- Symptoms are relieved by carbohydrate.

Symptoms

Neuroglycopenia

- Symptoms are **headache,** dizziness, depression, drowsiness, mental or neurologic impairment, visual disturbances, **craving** for sweets or caffeine.

Hyperadrenalism

- Symptoms are nervousness, irritability, trembling, sweating, tachycardia, insomnia, weakness.

FASTING HYPOGLYCEMIA

Etiology

- Blood sugar maintenance fails when meals are missed or during sleep. Symptoms most often indicate neuroglycopenia.

- Possible causes include
  1. oversecretion of insulin by tumor or hyperplastic beta cells
  2. insufficient hepatic glycogen due to carbohydrate restriction or storage defect
  3. defect in mobilization of hepatic glycogen due to endocrine or liver disorder (including that caused by alcoholism)

Clinical Signs

- Fasting plasma glucose levels are at least 10 mg/dL below laboratory normal values, accompanied by symptoms that are relieved by carbohydrate ingestion.
- Inappropriately high insulin levels at time of low glucose levels suggest an insulin-producing tumor.
- Fasting for up to 72 hours is required to identify borderline cases.

REACTIVE (POSTPRANDIAL, FUNCTIONAL) HYPOGLYCEMIA

Note: Symptoms following meals cannot be consistently shown to coincide with low plasma glucose in many cases. Some authorities have suggested that this condition be renamed **idiopathic postprandial syndrome.**

Subtypes and Clinical Pictures

Symptoms, usually suggesting **hyperadrenalism** (adrenergic response to declining blood glucose), occur within 5 hours after eating.

Alimentary Hypoglycemia

- Insulin overproduction is stimulated by rapid absorption of glucose from the gastrointestinal tract due to gastrectomy, overeating, or other causes.
- Symptoms tend to occur 1 to 3 hours after eating.
- Oral glucose/insulin tolerance test confirms the diagnosis if symptoms correlate.

Diabetic Hypoglycemia

- Normal insulin response is delayed, producing peak insulin levels later than peak glucose levels.
- Symptoms tend to occur 3 to 5 hours after eating.
- Early postprandial glucose values tend to be elevated.
- Oral glucose/insulin tolerance test confirms the diagnosis if symptoms correlate.
- Diabetic hypoglycemia is considered indicative of high risk to subsequent development of non-insulin–dependent diabetes. Other risk factors (family history, obesity) may be apparent.

Idiopathic Hypoglycemia

- Symptoms develop 1 to 5 hours after eating but may not coincide with low plasma glucose.
- Plasma epinephrine levels are usually elevated above 250 pg/mL in symptomatic patients.
- Oral glucose tolerance test often cannot distinguish these cases from asymptomatic controls.
- Rule out food allergy. See Chapter 7, "Food Allergy."

Other Causes

- Oversecretion of insulin may be caused by tumor or hyperplastic beta cells as in "Fasting Hypoglycemia" (above).

MANAGING HYPOGLYCEMIA

- **High-protein,** low-carbohydrate diets have been used successfully but are hazardous for long-term use.
- **Diabetic diet** plan appears to be beneficial in hypoglycemia. See Chapter 6, "Diabetes Mellitus."
  1. high-soluble-fiber, high-complex-carbohydrate diet
  2. diet low in sugar, other high glycemic response foods, and alcohol
  3. guar gum or pectin with meals if necessary
- Frequent meals or **snacks** may be necessary in fasting and alimentary hypoglycemias.
- Strict adherence to diet for 4 to 6 weeks should bring relief, but 3 months' adherence is optimal.
- After 3 months, liberalization of diet may include natural sources of simple sugars at first, eaten with regular meals to slow uptake. Eventually, severe cases can tolerate one high-sugar meal per week.
- **Chromium,** 200 mg/d, improved symptoms and reduced hypoglycemic responses to glucose in one study.

15. Immunity

BACKGROUND

Immune function may be understood as two inter-related systems, inborn immunity and adaptive immunity.

Inborn (Nonspecific) Immunity

- Inborn immunity involves natural **barriers** to infection—skin, mucous membranes, cilia, mucus, etc.
- Inborn immunity involves the **inflammatory response,** which attracts immune proteins and phagocytes (eg, monocytes, neutrophils, basophils) to areas of tissue injury. It is effective in killing bacteria but if prolonged will result in further tissue damage by inflammatory byproducts.

Adaptive (Specific) Immunity

- Macrophages that encounter bacteria present antigen to T lymphocytes, which then contribute additional inflammatory agents and activate proliferation of T and B lymphocytes.
- Antibody-mediated immunity: B lymphocytes, when activated, differentiate into plasma cells that produce specific antibodies belonging to several classes of immunoglobulins, ie, IgA, IgG, IgM, IgD, and IgE.
- Cell-mediated immunity: T lymphocytes, when activated, divide into several types of cells that either have direct cytotoxic effects

against foreign cells or produce substances (eg, interleukin, interferon) that help regulate other aspects of the immune response.

VERY-LOW-CALORIE INTAKE

- Very-low-calorie intake is associated with reduced stores of all nutrients required by the immune system, resulting in reduction in cell-mediated and antibody-mediated immunity and increased susceptibility to infection.

OBESITY

- Obesity is associated with increased frequency of infections and more fatalities from infections.
- Specific associations include reduced cellular immunity and high rates of iron and zinc deficiency (see below).

CARBOHYDRATE

- Excessive sugar intake may impair cell-mediated immunity and phagocytic function.

FATS

- Excess omega-6 polyunsaturated fatty acids (linoleic and arachidonic acid) suppress spleen function, increase likelihood of tumorigenesis in animals, and may reduce many aspects of immunity in humans, primarily through production of immunosuppressive prostaglandins. See Appendix A, "Prostaglandins and Related Eicosanoids."

- Medium-chain saturated fats (eg, coconut oil) and omega-3 fatty acids (eg, fish oils, linseed oil) reduce arachidonic acid levels, preventing overproduction of immunosuppressive prostaglandins.
- Fish oils fed to animals with burns or septicemia result in improved cell-mediated immunity and clinical outcome. Animals with autoimmune disorders fed fish oils demonstrate reductions in some indices of immune function. Current human studies employ 10 to 20 g/d.

PROTEIN, AMINO ACIDS, AND NUCLEOTIDES

- Protein deficiency, while relatively uncommon in free-living humans, reduces antibody production and T-cell activity.
- Conditions of high physiologic stress such as infection or widespread inflammation result in an increase in protein requirements up to 2.5 g/kg of body weight per day.
- Inflammatory conditions require large quantites of amino acids for visceral protein synthesis, wound healing, and immune system functions.
- **Branched-chain amino acids** supply fuel and stimulate protein synthesis during periods of physiologic stress. Up to 1 g/kg of body weight per day is beneficial.
- Supplemental **arginine** increases cellular immunity and enhances immune response in burned and traumatized patients. Up to 200 mg/kg of body weight per day parenterally or 15 to 30 g/d orally may be beneficial.
- Supplemental **glutamine** improves protein balance in stressed patients, especially those with intestinal pathology. Up to 500 mg/kg of body weight per day parenterally may be beneficial.
- Supplementary **nucleotides** (eg, ribonucleic acid) have been shown to boost cellular immunity and antibody production in animals. Current human studies utilize doses of 1500 to 2000 mg/d of yeast RNA, for example.

VITAMIN A

- Vitamin A supports many immune system functions as well as tissue resistance to infection.
- Vitamin A has an important role in **cancer resistance** and a possible role in cancer treatment.
- Improved immune function may be achieved with short-term doses of 300,000 IU or more of **retinol,** but impairment of immune function has also been reported at high doses.
- **Beta carotene,** 180 mg/d for 1 week, increased helper T-cell numbers. Other studies using 15 to 60 mg/d showed similar, dose-dependent effects.

VITAMIN B COMPLEX

- Folic acid and vitamin B12 deficiency impairs neutrophil function.
- Vitamin B6 deficiency diminishes antibody and lymphocyte activity.

VITAMIN C

- Deficiency impairs phagocyte function and cellular immunity.
- A dose of 1000 mg/d increases some parameters of immune response.
- Intramuscular injections improved immune response in some elderly subjects.

VITAMIN D

- Preliminary research suggests a regulatory effect of active vitamin D hormone on the immune system.

- Deficiency was associated with reduced immune responses in elderly men which reversed with oral supplemental vitamin D.

ANTIOXIDANTS

- Antioxidants appear to reduce cell damage during phagocytosis and inflammation.
- Vitamin E protects immune cell membranes. Vitamin E, 800 IU/d, improved immune response in healthy elderly persons.
- Caution: Excessive vitamin E (over 1000 IU/d) may reduce cell-killing ability.
- Zinc and copper function in intracellular antioxidant systems.
- Selenium deficiency may be immunosuppressive; 400 to 1000 µg/day may stimulate the immune system. There is one report of adverse effects at very high doses.

IRON

- Reduced iron nutrition results in proportionally more infections in children.
- Iron deficiency causes depressed cellular immunity.
- Caution: Excess iron may nourish microbes and depress some aspects of immune function.

ZINC

- Zinc is required for immunoprotein synthesis.
- Zinc plays specific roles in antibody response, natural killer cell activity, helper T-cell production, lymphocyte mobility, and tissue healing.
- Deficiency is associated with

1. thymus defects and atrophy
2. reduced lymphocyte count, especially T cells and natural killer cells with an increase in T suppressor cells
3. defects in phagocyte function
4. reduced immunoglobulins and antibody response
5. increased susceptibility to infections
6. delayed wound healing

- AIDS patients and many cancer patients often have reduced serum zinc levels.
- A dose of 100 mg/d has improved immune function in a group of healthy elderly persons.
- Caution: Zinc, 300 mg/d for 6 weeks, decreased lymphocyte responsiveness.

TRACE MINERALS

- Iodine deficiency, while uncommon in the US, is associated with decreased lymphocyte and neutrophil function.
- Copper deficiency is associated with increased incidence of infection and impaired cell-mediated immunity.

MISCELLANEOUS SUBSTANCES

- Excessive alcohol intake is detrimental to immune function.
- **Dimethylglycine,** 120 mg/d, resulted in a fourfold increase in antibody response in humans.
- Animal studies suggest that **germanium** may stimulate the immune system and inhibit tumors.

16. Indigestion

INCIDENCE

- There is a 25% incidence; indigestion is the second most common nutritional complaint (after weight problems).
- Indigestion is twice as common among men than among women.
- Peak age group for indigestion is 25 to 44 years.

CLINICAL ASSESSMENT

Location

- retrosternal, epigastric, right upper quadrant, diffuse upper abdomen, diffuse lower abdomen, referred pain to back

Quality

- bloating, belching, burning/cramping pain, nausea, flatulence, altered stool

Ominous Signs

- acute severity
- fever
- palpable masses
- bleeding

- severe tenderness
- jaundice
- progressive worsening

Offending Foods

Evaluate food/symptom history for repeated intolerance to any of the following common offenders:

- fat, protein (maldigestion)
- milk products (lactose intolerance, allergy)
- wheat, rye, barley, oats (gluten intolerance)
- beans, cabbage, onion, peppers, melons, other gas formers
- other frequently consumed foods

DIFFERENTIAL DIAGNOSIS

Rule Out Pathology

- hiatal hernia
- ulcer
- pancreatic disease
- gallbladder disease
- inflammatory bowel disease
- parasitic infection
- cancer

Eating Habits

- too fast
- too much

- under stress
- swallowing air

Irritation (Gastritis)

- spices
- alcohol
- acids
- drugs, other chemicals

Food Sensitivities

- allergy (See Chapter 7, "Food Allergy.")
- nonallergic intolerances (See Chapter 8, "Food Intolerance.")

Maldigestion (see below)

- low gastric hydrocholoric acid production (hypochlorhydria)
- pancreatic enzyme insufficiency
- biliary insufficiency
- intestinal lactase insufficiency (See "Simple Sugars" in Chapter 33, "Carbohydrates.")

Bacterial Flora Disorder (see below)

SECONDARY EFFECTS OF MALDIGESTION

- nutritional deficiency via related malabsorption or avoidance of food
- systemic allergy due to immunologic sensitization to incompletely digested food components

HYPOCHLORHYDRIA

Clinical Features

- protein intolerance, early (under 2 hours) postprandial distress
- contributing factors: increasing age, marijuana use
- associated with pernicious anemia or atopic or autoimmune disease
- increases susceptibility to
  1. deficiency of protein, folic acid, and most minerals
  2. iron-deficiency anemia
  3. bacterial gut infection
  4. pancreatic insufficiency
  5. reflux esophagitis
- verifiable through gastric analysis by intubation or telemetry (Comprehensive stool analysis may reveal undigested meat fibers.)

Nutrition Therapies

- Decrease protein portions at each meal.
- Consider **predigested protein** supplement or amino acid blend if deficient.
- Hypochlorhydria may be aggravated by zinc deficiency.
- Consider **betaine** or **glutamic** acid hydrochloride replacement supplement.
  1. Encapsulated powder is preferred over tablets.
  2. Consider 10 to 50 grain (500 to 2500 mg) per meal dose range.
  3. Gradually increase from minimal dose until symptoms respond or stomach discomfort occurs.
  4. Supplement is contraindicated in active ulcer or if causes burning pain.
  5. Supplement is contraindicated with prostaglandin inhibitor drugs (aspirin, ibuprofen, cortisone, other antiarthritis drugs).

PANCREATIC INSUFFICIENCY

Clinical Features

- fat and protein intolerance, delayed (1 to 4 hours) postprandial distress
- may have steatorrhea with normal stool color
- contributing factor: high alcohol intake
- associated with history of diabetes or hypochlorhydria
- increases susceptibility to
  1. deficiency of protein and fat-soluble vitamins
  2. pernicious anemia
  3. colonic bacterial overgrowth
  4. zinc deficiency
  5. food allergies (controversial)
- may be confirmed by depressed serum trypsin levels (Comprehensive stool analysis may reveal undigested fat, protein, and vegetable fibers.)

Nutrition Therapies

- Reduce dietary fat with smaller, more frequent, protein portions.
- Consider **predigested protein** supplement or amino acid blend if deficient.
- Consider **emulsified**/micellized/water-soluble **vitamin A** or E if deficient.
- Pancreatic insufficiency may be aggravated by zinc deficiency.
- Replacement is essential in cystic fibrosis and pancreatitis and after pancreatectomy.
- Consider optimal replacement **enzyme** products:
  1. noncoated more effective than enteric-coated
  2. pancreatin superior to bromelain or papain enzymes
  3. freeze-dried or azeotropic processing superior to other forms

- Potency labeling varies among manufacturers:
    1. 3X, 4X, 5X, etc. mean triple potency, quadruple potency, quintuple potency, etc.
    2. Total enzyme activity units multiplied by milligrams of given potencies are bases for product comparisons.
    3. Better products have individual batch potencies reported on label.
- Consider dosage range of two to eight tablets of average potency (300 mg, 4X).
- Oral enzymes are contraindicated in duodenal ulcer.

BILIARY INSUFFICIENCY

Clinical Features

- fat intolerance, early or delayed postprandial distress
- intolerance to gas-forming foods (see above)
- steatorrhea with light-colored stools if severe
- right upper quadrant tenderness or pain
- increases susceptibility to
    1. fat-soluble vitamin deficiencies
    2. elevated serum cholesterol
    3. constipation
    4. cholelithiasis and cholecystitis

Contributing Factors

- family history of gallbladder disease, Jewish heritage, obesity, female gender, perimenopausal age, fair complexion, multiparity, oral contraceptive use, possibly food allergies

- diets high in calories, sugar, fat, cholesterol
- diets low in fiber
- alcohol overconsumption, liver toxin overload
- deficiency of vitamins B6, B12, C, and E; folic acid; copper; sulfur; amino acids; essential fatty acids
- impaired/insufficient synthesis of lipotropic factors (phospholipids, choline, etc.)

Nutrition Therapies

- Reduce dietary saturated fat and cholesterol.
- Restrict hydrogenated fat.
- Correct related deficiencies, if present.
- Rule out food allergies.
- Botanicals: Beet leaf, Russian black radish, and other plants contain lipotropic precursors.
- Consider **taurine** which is required for bile salt synthesis.
- **Bile salts,** 50- to 100-mg dose per meal, may relieve symptoms and increase bile acid pool size. They are contraindicated in active ulcer or liver disease.
- **Lecithin,** 1- to 2-g dose per meal, may act as a substitute for bile salts.
- Animal research suggests that phosphatidyl choline, 10 g/d, may help solubilize bile.
- Biliary purge using olive oil to induce forceful expulsion of gallbladder contents has been advocated but may be dangerous.

COLONIC BACTERIAL FLORA DISORDERS

Colonic bacterial floral disorders are also known as toxic bowel syndrome and colonic bacterial hyperproliferation.

Clinical Features

- lower bowel discomfort, flatulence, constipation/diarrhea, foul-smelling stools; possibly systemic symptoms as well
- positive urinary indican test, indicating presence of systemic byproducts of putrefaction in colon
- may increase risk of colon cancer

Contributing Factors

- Previous antibiotic therapy increases risk of disruption of normal intestinal ecology.
- High-protein, low-fiber diet may encourage proliferation of putrefactive bacteria.
- Impaired protein digestion may result in malabsorbed proteins entering colonic environment.
- Prolonged intestinal transit time (normal considered to be below 72 hours) encourages growth of pathogenic anaerobes.

Nutrition Therapies

- Normalize **protein** intake.
- Restore normal digestion (see above).
- Improve transit time with increased intake of insoluble **fiber** and water, and exercise.
- Reinoculate with **acidophilus** culture.

Acidophilus Therapy

- Food sources include cultured dairy products (yogurt, kefir, cultured buttermilk), sweet acidophilus milk, pickled foods, sauerkraut.

- Commercial **culture supplements**
  1. contain viable organisms in high concentration (billions per gram)
  2. have a reasonable shelf-life (many require dark glass bottles, no fillers or capsules, refrigeration)
  3. are resistant to acid and bile
  4. have proven competitiveness with potential pathogens
- **Lactobacillus bifidus cultures** are recommended as normal flora supplements for infants and young children.

17. Kidney Stones

ETIOLOGY

- Over half of all stones are composed primarily of calcium oxalate. Calcium phosphate is also a common constituent.
- Uric acid stones are associated with gout.
- Cystine stones are associated with congenital cystinuria.
- Magnesium ammonium phosphate stones are associated with chronic bacterial infections.

RISK FACTORS FOR CALCIUM OXALATE STONES

- low water intake
- high urinary oxalate
- high urinary calcium
- diet high in meat, sugar, caffeine
- vitamin C intake over 6 g/d
- consumption of foods high in oxalate
    1. cocoa, tea, draft beer
    2. rhubarb, dark leafy greens
    3. beans, beets
    4. berry fruits, nuts
    5. wheat germ

MANAGEMENT OF CALCIUM OXALATE STONES

- Advise drinking **water** to cause 2 to 3 qt of urine per day (specific gravity less than 1.015).

- Maintain acid urine with intake of **cranberry,** plum/prune, or ascorbic acid.
- Consider diet low in meat, sugar, caffeine, and oxalate.
- Consider low calcium intake only if hypercalciuric.
- Consider **magnesium,** 300 mg/d.
- Consider vitamin B6, 150 mg/d.

MANAGEMENT OF OTHER STONES

Uric Acid Stones

- Advise water as above.
- Treat for gout. See "Gout" in Chapter 2, "Arthritis."
- Maintain alkaline urine with sodium bicarbonate.

Cystine Stones

- Advise water as above.
- Consider low-protein diet.
- Maintain alkaline urine with sodium bicarbonate.

18. Migraine Headache

BACKGROUND

Description

- chronic periodic head pain, usually unilateral, with vertigo, nausea and vomiting, photophobia, and/or "flashes of light"

Etiology

- Triggers cause catecholamine release, platelet aggregation, release of serotonin, and vasoconstriction.
- Resulting cerebral ischemia produces rebound vasodilation of arteries supplying the cranium.
- Migraine is related to atopy, an inherited imbalance in autonomic nervous system control resulting in inappropriate release of neurotransmitter substances.

Incidence

- Migraine afflicts at least 10% of the US population, mostly in young adulthood.
- Migraine is influenced by many risk factors (see below).
- Migraine is three to four times more common in females; it frequently occurs during menstruation.
- A significant percentage of migraine attacks (5% to 25%) may be due in whole or in part to dietary factors, including food hypersensitivity and hypoglycemia.

CLINICAL ASSESSMENT

Clinical assessment for migraine is facilitated by completing a migraine work sheet (Exhibit 18-1).

High-Risk Factors

- family history of migraine, sinus headache, other atopic diseases (asthma, hay fever, eczema, etc.)
- childhood history of gastrointestinal disturbances, motion sickness
- personal history of oral contraceptive use, perfectionistic personality

Migraine Triggers

- excessive stress—physical, chemical, or emotional
- exposure to glaring light, strong odors, other stimuli
- fatigue
- weather changes
- diet (see below)
- excessive vitamin A supplementation (at or above 25,000 IU)

Screen for Food Hypersensitivity

- Have patient keep food and symptom diary. Screen diet for the following:
  1. foods containing natural vasoactive chemicals that can initiate symptoms in 1½ to 12 hours
     (a) red wine and other alcoholic drinks
     (b) chocolate
     (c) aged cheese

Exhibit 18-1 Migraine Work Sheet

Circle appropriate findings
Symptoms
unilateral/bilateral head pain   vertigo   nausea   vomiting
photophobia   "flashes of light"   dizziness   drowsiness
anxiety   trembling   sweating

History
family history of migraine   other headaches   childhood gastric upsets
motion sickness   familial allergies   hay fever/sinusitis   asthma
eczema   history of low blood sugar   occurs during menstruation
occurs when stomach is empty   occurs after eating sweets
oral contraceptive use   vitamin A supplementation >20,000 U/d
excessive stress (describe)   perfectionistic personality   fatigue
exposure to glaring light   exposure to auto exhaust
sensitive to weather changes

Diet—How many times are the following eaten per week?

Natural or added chemicals
_____aged cheese   _____sour cream
_____red wine   _____imported wine
_____other alcoholic drinks   _____soft drinks
_____bacon/sausage   _____ham   _____liver
_____pork cold cuts (bologna, salami, etc.)
_____pickled herring   _____canned fish
_____chocolate   _____coffee/tea   _____cola
_____salty foods   _____MSG (Asian food, Accent, etc.)
_____french fries   _____salad bars   _____dried fruit
_____benzoic acid/sodium benzoate (preservative)
_____Yellow No. 5   _____yeast (breads, beer)

Possible migraine allergens
_____wheat   _____corn   _____milk   _____citrus
_____pineapple   _____grapes   _____coffee   _____tea
_____eggs   _____beef   _____pork   _____legumes
_____nuts   _____coconut   _____yeast   _____cola drinks

Hypoglycemic foods
_____desserts   _____candy   _____sugared soft drinks
_____sugared cereals   _____baked goods
_____added sugar   _____other sweets

(d) fermented sausage
   (e) sour cream
   (f) pickled herring
   (g) canned fish
2. additives with migraine-inducing potential
   (a) sodium (salty foods)
   (b) nitrites (cured meats)
   (c) monosodium glutamate (MSG)
3. known migraine allergens
   (a) wheat, corn, dairy products, citrus, pineapple, grapes, coffee, tea, chocolate
   (b) cane sugar, beef, pork, legumes, nuts, coconut, yeast, cola drinks

Screen for Hypoglycemia

- Screen food and symptom diary for migraine symptoms that occur between meals, especially when there are extended intervals between eating.
- See Chapter 14, "Hypoglycemia and Related Disorders."

PREVENTION AND TREATMENT

- Minimize occurrence of known triggers.
- Eliminate specific offending foods (there may be more than one). Often a restriction of *all* potential offenders must be recommended initially. If symptoms subside, foods may be added back one at a time while monitoring for relapses.
- Hypoglycemic individuals must maintain a low-sugar, high-complex-carbohydrate/high-dietary-fiber diet, possibly including several starchy between-meal snacks each day.
- A prostaglandin-modifying diet may help minimize platelet abnormalities (see Appendix A).

Nutrition Therapies

- **Fish oils,** 15 to 20 g/d, reduced frequency and severity in two controlled studies.

19. Muscle Cramps

Although many truly pathologic causes exist, such as hypoparathyroidism, vascular insufficiency, and various kinds of trauma, many complaints of muscle cramping have no obvious cause.

NON-NUTRITIONAL CAUSES

- Pay attention to the position of the patient when cramping occurs.
- A plantar-flexed foot while sleeping or exercising may set up a spasm of the calf muscle that occurs on further voluntary or involuntary contraction of the already shortened muscle. Women's high-heeled shoes are a problem for this reason.
- Passive stretching of the involved muscle is both a curative and preventative approach.

WATER AND ELECTROLYTES

- Muscle cramps during extensive exercising may be due simply to dehydration, in which case increasing water intake is effective.
- Mineral imbalances or deficiencies may contribute to muscle cramping. A relative lack of potassium, perhaps due to a diet high in salt and low in fresh fruits and vegetables, may impair local circulation, hasten fatigue, and increase irritability of muscle tissue.

THERAPEUTIC NUTRITION

- Increasing **magnesium** and even **calcium intake** has helped some individuals, especially pregnant women, reduce leg cramping.
- Older patients may complain of cramping that is due to vascular disorders such as atherosclerosis, intermittent claudication, or thrombophlebitis. Large doses of vitamin E may help some of these patients. See Chapter 5, "Cardiovascular Disorders."

20. Musculoskeletal Trauma

INFLAMMATORY PHASE

- Normal response to trauma for the first few days includes edema, release of inflammatory proteins, mobilization of leukocytes, and production of fibrin.
- Accumulation of cell debris, serum exudates, blood, and fibrin may impede healing by impairment of normal circulation.
- After therapeutic management of the trauma has begun, certain natural substances may be employed to speed healing.

Proteolytic Enzymes

- Proteolytic enzymes are derived from **bovine pancreas** (trypsin, chymotrypsin) or **pineapple** skin (bromelain).
- Proteolytic enzymes may reduce inflammatory response by breaking down **inflammatory proteins,** which cause vascular permeability and pain.
- Proteolytic enzymes may significantly improve local circulation by breaking down cell debris and fibrin prior to uptake by the lymphatic system.
- Absorption studies have demonstrated significant uptake of oral proteolytic enzymes through the gastrointestinal tract.
- Many studies have demonstrated the usefulness of proteolytic enzymes for various types of injury and inflammation.
- Prophylactic treatment of athletes with proteolytic enzymes resulted in fewer time-loss injuries and faster return to competition.

- Bromelain treatment of patients hospitalized for various injuries and inflammatory conditions resulted in 30% to 50% less time spent in the hospital than control patients.
- Treatment of patients with **lumbar disc prolapse** resulted in improved straight leg raising and decreased intake of analgesics.
- Despite promising clinical research, proteolytic enzymes are medically (Food and Drug Administration) approved only for **postepisiotomy pain** and swelling.
- Pharmaceutical-grade proteolytic enzymes are provided in enteric-coated tablets for protection through the upper gastrointestinal tract. The effectiveness of uncoated products is not known.
- Enzyme potencies are commonly defined in milk-clotting units (mcu). A given number of milligrams of products with similar potency should be equally effective.
- Bromelain in divided doses totaling 1200 mg/d of 2400 mcu potency between meals is in the upper range of typical protocols.
- Contraindications to the use of proteolytic enzymes include increased bleeding tendency, systemic infection, and allergy to food sources (ie, pineapple, pork, beef, papaya).

Bioflavonoids

- Bioflavonoids may significantly restrict vascular permeability to limit swelling.
- Bioflavonoids may inhibit inflammatory prostaglandins.
- Bioflavonoids are useful only before the peak of the inflammatory phase and will not reduce established edema.
- Prophylactic treatment of athletes with 600 to 1800 mg/d reduced healing time of injuries suffered by football players by two thirds in two studies.

Vitamin C

- Vitamin C was included in some positive animal studies in combination with **bioflavonoids.**
- Vitamin C may reduce free radical processes (with vitamin E) in inflamed tissues, may support **adrenal gland production** of anti-inflammatory hormones, and may have mild fibrinolytic and antihistamine effects.

PROLIFERATIVE PHASE

Regeneration of disrupted muscle and connective tissue requires the availability of appropriate protein and nonprotein precursors as well as nutrient cofactors required by synthesizing enzymes.

Wound Healing

- Research suggests that deficiencies of the following nutrients should be corrected to allow optimal tissue growth:
  1. calories, protein, essential fatty acids
  2. vitamins A, B1, B2, C, and E
  3. zinc, copper, manganese, and selenium.
- Trauma appears to increase requirements for protein (especially branched-chain amino acids) and vitamin C.
- Supplementations of **arginine,** glycine, proline, vitamins A and C, pantothenic acid, and zinc have each been associated with improved tissue healing.

Connective Tissue Repair

- Mucopolysaccharides (glycosaminoglycans, proteoglycans), the nonfibrous component of connective tissue, are composed of small amounts of protein, large amounts of specialized carbohydrates synthesized by chondrocytes and some minerals.
- Manganese is a required cofactor for the synthesis of mucopolysaccharides.
- Chondroitin sulfate and other mucopolysaccharide materials are available as supplements in the form of bovine tracheal extracts and mussel concentrates. Absorption in humans has been demonstrated. However, no direct studies of their effectiveness in human tissue healing have been reported.

Fracture Healing

- Nutritional considerations for tissue healing apply, as well, to the management of fractures. In addition, adequate dietary **calcium,** vitamin D, phosphorus, and magnesium further support remineralization.
- **Microcrystalline hydroxyapatite** has recently emerged as a possible improvement in the nutritional support of bone remineralization. Calcium absorption appears to be superior from this compound; studies have yielded promising results in the facilitation of fracture union. Six to eight grams per day is a typical therapeutic dose.

MUSCLE SPASM

The circumstances under which muscle spasm occurs help determine whether nutrition therapy will be of benefit.

- Protective muscle spasm resulting from strains and sprains is best managed with physical therapy. Oral supplements containing calcium, magnesium, and herbs such as valerian are popular treatments, but no clinical research has validated their usefulness in traumatic muscle spasm.
- Muscle cramps occurring without obvious trauma may have nutritional or non-nutritional causes. See Chapter 19, "Muscle Cramps."

21. Obesity

DEFINITIONS AND STANDARDS

Weight for Height

Height/Weight Tables

- 20% or more above upper limit of ideal = obese
- apply to adults over age 24 years
- need frame size assessment. See "Physical Tests" in Chapter 27, "History and Examination."

Body Mass Index

- body mass index (BMI) = (weight in kilograms)/(square of height in meters)
- 30 or greater = obese

Infant/Child Growth Charts

- above 90th percentile = obese

Body Fat Percentage

Triceps Plus Subscapular Skinfold Thicknesses

- above 85th percentile or
  1. over 45 mm in men = obese
  2. over 65 mm in women = obese

Measured by Hydrostatic Weight, Bioelectric Impedance, or Other Methods

- see "Physical Tests" in Chapter 27, "History and Examination"
- above 24% in men = obese
- above 33% in women = obese

INCIDENCE

- Depending on definition, 12% to 30% of US population are obese. Many more are overweight, yet below obesity standards.

UNUSUAL CAUSES

- rare genetic disorders
- endocrinopathies—Cushing's syndrome, hyperinsulinism, hypothyroidism
- drugs—cyproheptadine, tricyclic antidepressants, phenothiazines

HEALTH RISKS

- Truncal (male pattern) obesity appears to be more dangerous than pelvic (female pattern) obesity.

Mortality

- gradual increase with overweight in males
- sudden increase at 45% above ideal weight for females

Morbidity

- possibly the key to mortality
- possibly atherosclerosis and related diseases although obese individuals who do *not* develop hypertension, hyperlipidemia, and/or diabetes may not have increased risk from obesity alone
- diabetes—doubled risk for every 20% above ideal body weight; affects insulin sensitivity
- hypertension—highest risk in adult-onset obesity and obesity in small-framed individuals
- gallbladder disease—especially middle-aged women
- hormone-dependent cancers—especially endometrial cancer
- colon cancer—men only
- gynecologic disorders—menstrual irregularity, polycystic ovaries and infertility
- pregnancy complications—hypertension, toxemia, abnormal labor
- osteoarthritis and gout

BIOLOGIC AND ENVIRONMENTAL MECHANISMS

Much remains to be understood about the mechanisms of obesity development. The following factors each play roles of greater or lesser importance.

Genetic Influences

- obesity risk according to parental obesity
  1. neither parent obese—10% risk
  2. one parent obese—40% risk
  3. both parents obese—80% risk
- endomorph somatotype—soft, round body; wide costal angle, wide pubic angle
- gynecoid (pelvic) versus android (truncal) obesity (see above)

Developmental Influences—Fat Cell Size and Number

Hyperplastic/Hypercellular Obesity

- Cell number can normally increase only in infancy and (in females) in adolescence.
- Hyperplastic obesity is controlled by genetics, at least in part.
- Excess calories may stimulate fat cell number increases during these periods.

Hypertrophic Obesity

- 90% to 95% of obesity incidence
- usually adult onset
- associated with highest mortality and morbidity risks

Appetite Regulation

Hypothalamic Controls

- lateral hypothalamus—feeding center, primary drive for appetite
- ventromedial hypothalamus—satiety center, inhibits luteinizing hormone
- neurotransmitter signals received by hypothalamus:
  1. mediated by dopamine, norepinephrine, serotonin, acetylcholine
  2. α-adrenergic—feeding stimulus
  3. β-adrenergic—satiety stimulus
  4. dopaminergic—satiety stimulus
- satiety also caused by brain endorphins and enkephalins

Influences on Hypothalamus

Metabolic Factors. How does the brain know when fuel stores are low?
- glucostatic control theory—appetite is mediated by serum glucose and/or insulin levels
  1. short- and medium-range control
- lipostatic control theory—appetite is mediated by glycerol or free fatty acid levels
  1. long-range control
  2. possible basis for set-point control of adipose cell size
- aminostatic control theory—appetite is mediated directly or through fluctuations in neurotransmitter levels
- thermostatic control theory—appetite is mediated by thermogenic effect of food

Hormone Signals.
- Insulin, glucocorticoids, thyroid hormones, estrogen, and gastrointestinal hormones have varying effects on appetite.

Gastrointestinal Signals.
- Stretch receptors in gastrointestinal tract detect presence of food and stimulate vagus nerve.
- Most gut peptides cause satiety—cholecystokinin, bombesin, thyrotropin-releasing hormone, somatostatin.

Sensory Signals.
- Taste and smell have direct effects on appetite.

Psychologic/Social Stimuli.
- Pleasant and unpleasant emotions have varying effects on appetite.

Neurobiochemical Factors.
- Dopamine drugs such as amphetamine and phenylpropanolamine inhibit appetite.
- Endorphins apparently inhibit appetite.

Exercise Effects.
- Physically active people appear to have appetite more in tune to actual body needs than do sedentary ones.

Environmental/Psychologic Factors—Appetite Not Involved

- Emotional disorders may lead to increased eating—binge eating, bulemia, night-eater syndrome.
- Social occasions may encourage eating regardless of appetite.
- Distracted eating, such as in front of television, may increase intake regardless of appetite.
- Variety in diet encourages overeating, even in animals.

Intrinsic Food Factors

- So-called "empty calorie" foods containing additional sugar, fat, and/or alcohol allow for increased intake before satiety mechanisms are activated.
- High-fiber foods increase chewing time and activate stretch receptors in the stomach, allowing satiety to be achieved earlier.

Thermogenic Regulation—Controlling Energy Use

- Body heat is wasted energy and is a means of releasing unwanted calories.
- All of the energy transfers that occur during the burning of body fuels and lead to the formation and utilization of high-energy bonds are inefficient and result in energy loss as heat.
- Excess calories, exercise, and stress may stimulate increased wasting of energy by *futile cycles*.

- Futile cycles may include round trips through membranes, release and restorage of fuels, and initiation and reversal of glycolysis and oxidative phosphorylation.
- Genetic and acquired differences may exist in the ability to utilize thermal regulation to burn excess calories:
  1. Obese persons have 22% less sodium-potassium adenosinetriphosphatase activity.
  2. Higher percentage fat bodies need fewer calories to maintain same weight (less mitochondria in fat tissue).
  3. Hypothyroidism leads to obesity.

Brown Fat—Tissue Specializing in Futile Cycles (Controversial)

- occurs in limited amounts at various sites in the body
- contains larger, more numerous mitochondria
- produces heat as wasted energy by continuously breaking down and resynthesizing triglycerides
- is hypofunctional in genetically obese animals
- is stimulated by thyroid and adrenal hormones

Specific Dynamic Effect of Food

- Fat requires the least (4%) energy to be processed; protein requires the most (15 to 30%).
- Eating increases body heat production to varying degrees in different people—probably a genetic trait.
- Carbohydrates, polyunsaturated fatty acids, and fructose appear to stimulate thermogenesis compared to protein, saturated fat, and sucrose.
- Caffeine, up to 200 mg/d, is thermogenic and lipolytic.

Specific Dynamic Effect of Exercise

- Exercise not only burns calories but may increase metabolic rate up to several hours afterward in the short run as well as more permanently through increasing lean body mass.

Specific Dynamic Effect of Stress

- Catecholamines and other sympathetomimetic agents (ephedrine) stimulate heat production in certain tissues.

WEIGHT LOSS THERAPEUTICS

- See Chapter 26, "Weight Loss and Weight Control."

22. Osteoporosis

DESCRIPTION

- Osteoporosis is a reduction in bone mass. Bone loss is especially serious in spine, femoral neck, and distal radius, which are then predisposed to fracture.
- Postmenopausal osteoporosis affects women aged 50 to 65 years.
- Senile osteoporosis affects both sexes over age 75 years.

INCIDENCE AND DEMOGRAPHICS

- Osteoporosis affects approximately 25% of all women, 16% of men.
- At least 10% of all individuals over age 50 years are highly prone to fractures.
- About 6 million spontaneous fractures due to osteoporosis occur annually in the United States at a cost of $1 billion and a mortality rate of 15%.

CLINICAL ASSESSMENT

Major High-Risk Factors

- osteoporosis in family history
- light-skinned, small-frame female gender
- long postmenopausal life expectancy
- sedentary life style

- low calcium intake
- low vitamin D status
- risk factors may be assessed by questionnaire (Exhibit 22-1)

Associated Risk Factors

- high dietary protein, phosphorus, fiber, salt, alcohol, caffeine
- smoking
- stress
- frequent weight-loss dieting
- no full-term pregnancies and no oral contraceptive use
- medications: antacids (except calcium carbonate), corticosteroids, thyroid, tetracycline, some diuretics and anticonvulsants
- diseases: hyperparathyroidism, hyperthyroidism, Cushing's syndrome, kidney disease, diabetes, rheumatoid arthritis, periodontal disease, achlorhydria, malabsorption syndromes
- excessive supplemental retinol or vitamin D
- risk factors may be assessed by questionnaire (Exhibit 22-1)

Laboratory Tests

- Laboratory tests possibly are useful to determine the rate of bone loss at a given time.
- Serum total calcium will be normal but serum ionized calcium may be high-normal or elevated.
- Fasting urinary calcium/creatinine ratio over 0.4 is correlated with osteoporotic bone loss in the absence of gross bone or kidney pathology.
- Fasting urinary hydroxyproline/creatinine ratio is considered a good clinical index of bone resorption in the absence of gross bone or kidney pathology.

Exhibit 22-1 Osteoporosis Risk Factor Questionnaire

Have you been told you have osteoporosis or "thinning bones"?	YES	NO
Have you experienced a decrease in height and/or rounding or humping of the upper back?	YES	NO
Have you ever had a spontaneous fracture (not caused by a major traumatic event) of the hip, wrist, or back?	YES	NO
Do any of the above questions apply to any of your older female blood relatives?	YES	NO
Have you experienced menopause either naturally or through surgery?	YES	NO
If so, how many years ago?		_____
Are you taking female hormones regularly?	YES	NO
What is your age?		_____
your race?		_____
your height?		_____
your present weight?		_____
Has your weight varied greatly from this amount during your adult life?	YES	NO
If it has, please describe _____		

Do you have a small body size (wear petite-size clothes)?	YES	NO
How many times per *week* do you eat the following portions of food?		
One cup of milk, buttermilk, yogurt, milk puddings or custards (300 mg calcium each)		_____
One-half cup (one scoop) ice cream/ice milk (100)		_____
One-half cup cottage cheese (50–75)		_____
Two slices hard cheese (200)		_____
One-quarter package (3 1/2 oz) tofu (soybean curd) (150)		_____
Do you take calcium supplements regularly?	YES	NO
If so, how many milligrams per day?		_____
How many minutes per *week* do you spend outdoors in direct sunlight with at least your face and hands exposed?		_____
Do you take a supplement containing vitamin D?	YES	NO

(continues)

Exhibit 22-1 Continued

How many cups (8 oz) of milk or milk-containing products
do you use per *week*? (100 IU vitamin D each)   _____

How many hours per *week* do you spend *on your feet* walking,
exercising, or working at a moderate or heavy level?   _____

Indicate which of the following statements applies to you, or that has applied
to you in the past. (YES answers indicate increased risk)

YES or NO

_____ You DO eat a lot of protein foods

_____ You DO eat a lot of packaged convenience foods

_____ You DO eat a lot of high-fiber foods

_____ You DO drink carbonated soft drinks regularly

_____ You DO drink four or more cups of coffee per day

_____ You DO use and enjoy salt and salty foods

_____ You DO smoke a pack of cigarettes or more per day

_____ You DO drink more than one alcoholic drink per day or seven total per week

_____ You ARE under an excessive amount of stress

_____ You DO take antacids regularly

_____ You HAVE NEVER used birth control pills

_____ You DO take corticosteroid, anticonvulsant, thyroid or diuretic medications

_____ You DO take over 5000 IU of vitamin A in a daily supplement

_____ You DO take over 1000 IU of vitamin D in a daily supplement

_____ You DO go on a diet to lose weight often

_____ You HAVE been told you have one of the following conditions (circle which one)

hyperparathyroidism   hyperthyroidism   Cushing's syndrome
kidney disease   diabetes   rheumatoid arthritis
periodontal (gum) disease   achlorhydria (deficient stomach acid)

_____ You HAVE had surgical removal of part of the stomach (gastrectomy)

_____ You HAVE NOT had any full-term pregnancies

Bone Density Studies

- Bone density studies are useful for determining the amount of bone present at a given time.
- Routine radiographs are of limited value until the disease has progressed significantly and/or spontaneous fractures have occurred.
- Accurate assessment of bone density requires tomographic densitometry or photon absorptiometry techniques.

PREVENTION

- Minimization of all risk factors that are modifiable (see above) is the cornerstone of osteoporosis prevention. This should be addressed in young patients as well as older ones.
- High-risk individuals appear to require 1200 to 1500 mg of calcium per day. Dairy products and tofu are the best sources and provide 100 to 300 mg per serving, but this may not be sufficient. Supplementation is recommended.
- Vitamin D deficiency may occur in older individuals. Adequate exposure to sunlight, ingestion of fortified milk, or supplementation should be implemented.
- Weight-bearing exercise on a daily basis will reduce and perhaps reverse bone loss.
- Vitamin K, 1 mg/d, in one study reduced calcium and hydroxyproline excretion in postmenopausal women.
- Boron as a trace element may be important in hardening bone.

TREATMENT

Existing osteoporosis may be slowed and possibly reversed through attention to the factors mentioned above with the following modifications and additions:

- **Calcium therapy** is sometimes effective at levels of 1000 to 3000 mg/d. Effectiveness is most apparent after the fifth postmenopausal year. Additional broad vitamin/mineral supplementation may be beneficial as well.
- **Vitamin D** therapy at levels above 400 IU may give added benefit. In resistant cases, active 1,25-dihydroxyvitamin D3 hormone (by prescription) may be more effective.
- **Weight-bearing exercise** therapy must consider the skeletal and aerobic fitness of the elderly patient.
- **Microcrystalline hydroxyapatite,** 6 to 8 g/d as well as calcium citrate-malate, 1000 mg/d, reverses bone loss, according to preliminary studies.
- **Estrogen** replacement therapy has been shown to be effective in slowing down or reversing postmenopausal bone loss, especially in conjunction with calcium therapy. Many side effects exist, however, including increased risk of breast and uterine cancer.

23. Pregnancy, Lactation, and Infancy

PRECONCEPTION NUTRITION

Oral Contraceptives and Deficiencies

- Consider treating possible deficiencies associated with use of oral contraceptives:
  1. vitamin B6
  2. vitamin B12
  3. folic acid
  4. calcium
  5. phosphorus
  6. magnesium
  7. zinc
- Use of a broad-spectrum prenatal supplement by women attempting to conceive is recommended.

Pre-existing Diseases

- Control pre-existing conditions that cause high-risk pregnancy:
  1. diabetes
  2. hypertension
  3. anemia
  4. malabsorption
  5. underweight
  6. obesity
  7. substance abuse

Clinical Protocols 129

PREGNANCY WEIGHT GAIN GOALS

- Prepregnancy ideal body weight (IBW) and optimal weight gain during pregnancy are as follows:
  1. 90% IBW: 28 to 40 lb recommended gain
  2. 100% IBW: 25 to 35 lb recommended gain
  3. 120% IBW: 15 to 25 lb recommended gain
  4. 135% IBW: 15 lb recommended gain
- Women at high risk of producing small babies (African Americans, underweight, young adolescents) should aim for the upper end of the recommended ranges.
- Women of short stature (under 5 ft 2 in) should aim for the lower end of the recommended ranges.
- Women expecting twins should gain 35 to 45 lb in all cases.
- Weight gain for women at normal prepregnancy weight should approximate 3 to 4 lb total in the first trimester and 1 lb/wk during the second and third trimesters.
- Excessive weight gain may reflect water retention, in which case the patient should be closely monitored for preeclampsia or hypertension (see below).
- Caution: Excessive weight gain does not justify severe dietary restrictions that might interfere with normal nutrition.

INCREASED DIETARY NEEDS IN PREGNANCY

- Calorie needs increase 300 kcal/d during second and third trimesters.
- Protein needs increase 10 to 15 g/d over normal requirements, resulting in a requirement of 60 g/d for typical women.
- Diet should include at least four servings each of milk products, fruits/vegetables, and breads/cereals, plus two servings of meat/protein foods.
- Emphasize foods high in vitamin A, vitamin C, calcium, and iron.

- See Appendix H for complete *1989 Recommended Dietary Allowances*.

ESSENTIAL PRENATAL SUPPLEMENTS

- vitamin B6, 2 to 10 mg/d, to maintain normal serum levels
- folic acid, to ensure total intake of 400 to 800 µg/d
- calcium, to ensure total intake of 1200 mg/d
- iron, 30 to 60 mg/d, depending on iron status and diet (see below)
- vitamins D and B12 for strict vegetarians
- multiple vitamin/mineral supplements for smokers, alcohol and drug users, and other high-risk women
- zinc and copper if high-dose iron is prescribed for treating anemia

NUTRITIONAL EXCESSES TO AVOID

Limit the following to RDA levels (unless otherwise indicated):
- vitamin A—associated with birth defects
- vitamin B12 (megadoses)—may create dependency syndrome
- vitamin C (megadoses)—may increase risk of abortion, may create dependency syndrome
- vitamin D—may cause hypercalcemia
- iodine—associated with mental retardation and neonatal death

NUTRITIONAL CONSIDERATIONS IN COMMON PREGNANCY COMPLICATIONS

Miscarriage (Spontaneous Abortion)

- advise avoidance of smoking, alcohol, caffeine
- consider vitamin E, 200 IU/d if susceptible to miscarriage
- consider bioflavonoids, 600 mg/d if susceptible to miscarriage

Anemia of Pregnancy

- Order complete blood count at first visit and at beginning of each trimester. Ferritin levels will help identify high-risk patients in early pregnancy.
- Treat existing anemia with iron, 100 mg/d, and folic acid, 1000 mg/d.
- Monitor progress weekly with reticulocyte count until hematocrit and hemoglobin are normal.

Morning Sickness

The following protocol may bring relief in uncomplicated cases:
- dry toast or crackers in the morning
- small, frequent meals
- separate consumption of foods and liquids
- avoid cooking odors
- ginger root tea or powdered ginger root, 1 g/d
- vitamin B6, 75 to 600 mg/d
- vitamin K, 5 mg/d, with vitamin C, 25 mg/d (effective in one uncontrolled study)

Leg Cramps

- Consider calcium, 2000 mg/d.
- Advise avoidance of excess phosphorus (cola drinks, processed foods).

Pica

- Pica is a craving for non-food substances:
  1. clay
  2. dirt

3. laundry starch
  4. ice
  5. junk food?
- Pica may indicate anemia.

PREECLAMPSIA/ECLAMPSIA (TOXEMIA)

- Eclampsia is a major cause of maternal death.
- Monitor blood pressure: 30/15 mm Hg above usual is ominous.
- Monitor urinary protein.
- Monitor for edema/sudden weight gain.

Prevention

- Avoid pregnancy if more than 30% overweight.
- If obese, avoid weight gain over 4 lb/mo.

Nutritional Control

- Ensure an adequate diet; sodium should not be restricted.
- Consider vitamin B6, 10 mg/d (one uncontrolled study).
- Diuretics are useless and may be harmful.
- Consider calcium, 2000 mg/d if hypertension develops.

GESTATIONAL DIABETES

Risk Factors

- obesity
- abnormal prepregnancy glucose tolerance

- previous baby over 9 lb birth weight
- death or anomaly in previous fetus/neonate

Laboratory Monitoring

- High-risk: Monitor serum glucose at first visit after glucose challenge.
- Monitor all others at 6 months.
- Check regularly urinary glucose (may give false-positive results; confirmation by serum glucose testing is necessary).

Prevention

- Avoid pregnancy if more than 30% above standard weight.
- Avoid excessive weight gain (over 4 lb/mo during final 6 months) during pregnancy if obese. However, do not advise a low-calorie diet.
- Ensure adequate vitamin B6 and chromium.

Nutritional Control

- See Chapter 6, "Diabetes Mellitus," for general protocol.
- Consider vitamin B6, 100 mg/d.

PREVENTION OF ADVERSE PREGNANCY OUTCOMES

Fetal Mortality and Morbidity

- Avoid use of tobacco, alcohol, and other drugs.
- Prevent/control gestational diabetes, hypertension, and preeclampsia/eclampsia.

Congenital Anomalies

- Refer for medical advice on use of all prescription medications.
- Avoid more than four caffeine sources per day.
- Avoid alcohol and artificial sweeteners.
- Ensure adequate folic acid, zinc.

Prematurity

- Ensure adequate nutrition, especially protein, througout pregnancy.

Low Birth Weight

- Achieve adequate prepregnancy weight (not more than 10% below standards).
- Maintain adequate prenatal weight gain (over 2 lb/mo during last 6 months, total of 22 to 30 lb during entire term).
- Avoid smoking, alcohol, and other drugs.
- Ensure adequate iron, folic acid, zinc.

Mental Retardation

- Avoid alcohol and other drugs.

Pediatric Neurologic and Behavioral Problems

- Avoid alcohol and other drugs.

- Refer for medical advice on use of tranquilizers and amphetamines.

LACTATION

Prevent General Malnutrition

- Calorie needs increase 500 to 650 kcal/d during lactation, depending on maternal weight gain.
- Protein needs increase 15 g/d over normal during first 6 months of lactation, 12 g/d for second 6 months.
- Emphasize foods high in vitamin A and vitamin C.
- Consider supplements of calcium, magnesium, zinc, and iron.
- Avoid eating nonfood substances (pica).
- Ensure adequate fluid intake.
- See Appendix H for complete *1989 Recommended Dietary Allowances*.
- Refer for medical advice on use of prescription and nonprescription drugs.

Avoid Nutritional Excesses

- Large doses of vitamin B6 may suppress lactation.

Prevent Neurologic and Behavioral Problems

- Advise against consumption of alcohol, nicotine, marijuana, street drugs, and caffeine.
- Ensure adequate calories, protein, and weight gain during pregnancy.

INFANT NUTRITION

Encourage Breast-Feeding for As Long As Possible

- Breast-feeding provides immunoglobulins; is the most nutritionally balanced, safe, and easily digestible infant food; prevents bacterial overgrowth in colon; promotes maternal-infant bonding; and promotes normal mouth/jaw development.
- Infant supplements of vitamin D (400 IU/d), vitamin K (2 mg at birth), iron (7 mg/d if mother was anemic), and fluoride (0.25 mg/d if water supplies are low) are desirable.

Choose Appropriate Formulas When Necessary

- Plain cow's or goat's milk is not correctly balanced for infants and may be dangerous.
- Formulas should have digestible quality proteins or amino acids, essential fatty acids, balanced vitamin/mineral content, and appropriate electrolyte concentration.
- Protein source may be cow's milk, soy, or amino acid mix depending on infant's tolerance. Soy-based formulas are not recommended for premature infants.
- Carbohydrate source may be lactose, corn syrup, sucrose, maltose, or dextrins, depending on infant's tolerance.
- Fortification with tyrosine, cystine, taurine, and omega-3 fatty acids is desirable.
- Iron-fortified formula is indicated for anemic infants.
- Increased vitamin E content is indicated if formula contains high levels of polyunsaturated fat.
- Modified-fat formula is indicated in malabsorption syndromes.

Clinical Protocols 137

After Weaning, Begin to Build a Balanced and Varied Diet

- Place less emphasis on milk.
- Place more emphasis on meat and non-meat proteins, grain products, fruits, and vegetables.
- Use homemade foods whenever possible.
- Avoid foods high in salt, sugar, coarse fibers, or nitrates (beets, spinach, other greens).
- Do not over-restrict fat and cholesterol.
- Avoid common allergens: wheat, corn, egg white, cow's milk, peanuts, citrus, tomato, chocolate/cocoa.
- If certain food groups are rejected, they should be reintroduced later, provided as finger foods, and/or made more appealing in color, texture, or taste.

Ensure Optimal Nutrition, Especially in Low-Birth-Weight Infants

- Ensure adequate calories for growth and heat production.
- Ensure adequate protein for growth.
- Ensure adequate carbohydrate to maintain blood sugar.
- Ensure adequate fat and cholesterol for calories and hormone synthesis.
- Ensure adequate vitamins C, D, E, and K.
- Ensure adequate calcium, magnesium, iron, copper, and zinc.
- Avoid foods with too much sodium; maintain proper calcium/phosphorus ratio.
- See Appendix H for complete *1989 Recommended Dietary Allowances.*

Prevent Life-Threatening Imbalances

- Prevent dehydration with adequate fluids, moderate electrolyte intake, and prompt treatment of diarrhea, vomiting, and fever.

Monitor for Normal Weight Gain with Pediatric Growth Charts

- Changes in length and weight from month to month are useful nutritional indexes, but accuracy is usually better for weight measurements.
- Head circumference changes are not very useful for nutritional evaluation.
- Extremely high or low percentile rankings may be significant, as may sharp deviations from previous percentile rankings.

Maintain Normal Growth

- If significant overweight is present, check for overconcentrated formula, too frequent feedings, use of feeding for comfort or reward, or insufficient activity.
- Slowing of growth of length should not be allowed.
- If weight gain is insufficient, check for overdiluted formula, infrequent feedings, and gastrointestinal disorders.

Suspect Nutritional Deficiencies in Special Situations

- anemia if mother's iron status has been poor
- vitamin K deficiency if not supplemented at birth
- vitamin B12 deficiency if mother is a strict vegetarian
- fat-soluble vitamin deficiencies if malabsorption is present
- fluoride deficiency in low fluoride areas

Prevent/Control Food Allergies

- Advise exclusive breast-feeding for first 6 months. High-risk cases are advised to restrict major allergenic foods in the mother's diet. See Chapter 7, "Food Allergy."
- Use only hypoallergenic formula (containing protein hydrolysate) to supplement breast milk.
- Avoid cow's milk and solid foods for at least 6 months.
- Introduce new foods one at a time, adding least allergenic foods first, to allow for identification of potential allergies.
- Suspect food allergy if vomiting, colic, irritability, rashes, or frequent infections occur.

Monitor for Anemia Routinely

- Use hemoglobin or hematocrit to screen.
- Use MCV, ferritin, transferrin saturation, or protoporphyrin to confirm.
- Give iron supplement, 1 mg/kg, until blood values normalize.
- Hemoglobin/hematocrit should respond within 4 to 6 weeks.

Prevent Impaired Neurologic Development

- Ensure adequate calories, protein, and weight gain during first 6 months.
- Avoid artificial sweeteners in large amounts.
- Refined sugar restriction has not been proven to affect the behavior of the majority of hyperactive children in controlled studies.
- The Feingold diet, which eliminates all artificial flavors and colors, the preservatives butylated hydroxyanisole (BHA) and BHT, foods containing natural salicylates, and many over-the-counter medications, has failed to demonstrate consistent results in most

controlled studies. However, it is believed to be effective in approximately 2% of hyperactive children. In addition, a placebo effect is common.
- Megavitamin therapy has not been effective in controlling hyperactivity in most studies, although some children have responded to either niacin or pyridoxine.

Prevent Early Dental Caries

- Avoid allowing the infant to sleep with bottle in mouth.
- Avoid sweetened pacifiers.
- Avoid high-sugar liquids and solid food.
- Clean the infant's teeth regularly.
- Use fluoride supplements where necessary.

24. Premenstrual Syndrome

INCIDENCE

- Premenstrual syndrome affects about 40% to 50% of women in the reproductive years.
- There is a high correlation with job absenteeism, child abuse, and marital strife.

SYMPTOM CLASSIFICATION

- Symptoms typically appear after midcycle and improve or subside with menses.
- Symptoms of premenstrual tension (PMT) types A, H, C, and D are listed below from common to least common:

PMT-A

- anxiety, irritability, and nervous tension
- mood swings

PMT-H

- transient weight gain (more than 3 lb), edema
- abdominal bloating and tenderness
- breast congestion, mastalgia

PMT-C

- increased appetite
- craving for sweets
- indulgence usually followed by fainting, fatigue, palpitations, and/or headache

PMT-D

- depression
- withdrawal
- lethargy
- confusion
- suicidal thoughts

ETIOLOGY THEORIES

Impaired Estrogen Metabolism

- associated with low progesterone/17β-estradiol ratio and/or low estrogen quotient (estriol divided by the sum of estradiol and estrone)
- related to degree of adiposity due to excess estrogen production in adipose tissue
- due to decreased hepatic estrogen clearance, which is dependent on certain B-vitamins and magnesium
- due to increased estrogen deconjugation by intestinal bacteria, which is reversible with low-fat, high-fiber diets and, possibly, *Lactobacillus acidophilus* therapy

Abnormal Neuroendocrine Regulation

- serotonin insufficiency, which may respond to tryptophan and vitamin B6 therapy
- endorphin insufficiency, which may respond to aerobic exercise
- melatonin insufficiency, which may respond to increased exposure to full-spectrum light
- dopamine insufficiency, which may respond to tyrosine and vitamin B6 therapy
- prolactin excess, which may be inhibited by dopamine and prostaglandin (PG) E_1

Prostaglandin Imbalances

- increased PGE_2 and $PGF_{2\alpha}$
- decreased PGE_1
- may respond to appropriate precursor manipulation (see Appendix A)

Abnormal Glucose Metabolism

- may promote or be aggravated by premenstrual cravings
- may contribute to mood swings
- see Chapter 14, "Hypoglycemia and Related Disorders"

CLINICAL MANAGEMENT

Consider Pathologies

- Rule out psychologic disorders.
- Rule out disorders of kidney and endocrine function.
- Screen for alcoholism and mammary dysplasia.

Improve Diet and Life Style Factors

- Normalize weight.
- Exercise regularly.
- Limit total fats, emphasizing polyunsaturated fats.
- Emphasize vegetable proteins over animal proteins.
- Increase dietary fiber intake.
- Limit dietary simple carbohydrates.
- Limit dietary salt intake.
- Limit caffeine and other central nervous system stimulants.
- Limit use of alcohol and tobacco.
- Reduce stress, especially with meditation.

Provide Nutritional Therapies

- Consider **vitamin B6,** 100 to 600 mg/d, taken with smaller doses of the remaining vitamin B complex to reduce side effects. Advise patient on warning signs of peripheral neuropathy.
- Consider **magnesium,** 500 to 800 mg/d in well-absorbed form, taken away from high-calcium meals and supplements.
- Consider **vitamin E,** 100 to 400 IU/d, if breast pain is significant.
- Consider γ-linolenic acid, 240 to 320 mg/d, as **evening primrose oil,** black currant oil, or borage oil.

25. Sports Nutrition

GOALS OF THE ATHLETE'S DIET

- The athlete's diet should be compatible with long-term nutritional health goals of deficiency prevention and avoidance of hazardous excesses.
- Individual nutritional needs arising from pre-existing health problems and other abnormalities must be appreciated.
- Specific sports-related nutritional considerations must be made according to the nature of the particular activity and the availability of relevant information.

CALORIES

- Calorie requirements for training may be much greater than those for the nonathlete.
- Early fatigue, muscle tissue loss, and amenorrhea in women are associated with inadequate calorie intake.
- Energy requirements may be estimated from the following formula:

    (Kilograms ideal body weight × C) + exercise cost

    where C equals 30 for growing athletes and 24 for most adults. Exercise costs may be estimated from the following:

    Kilocalories expended hourly per kilogram body weight
Baseball: 4.1–5.3	Dancing: 3.6–4.8
Basketball: 6.0–8.5	Football: 7.3
Cycling: 4.8–9.7	Golf: 3.6–4.8

Handball: 8.5
Mountain climbing: 8.7
Rowing: 12.0
Running: 9.7–17.2
Skating: 4.8–8.7
Skiing, downhill: 8.5
Skiing, cross-country: 9.7

Soccer: 7.8
Swimming: 3.4–9.7
Tennis: 6.0–8.5
Volleyball: 4.8–8.5
Walking: 2.9–5.8
Wrestling: 11.1

Eating Disorders

- Eating disorders are common in certain athletes who are motivated to over-restrict calories in order to compete in lower weight categories or attain a more aesthetic body shape.
- Eating disorders will likely impair performance and may have dangerous side effects.
- See Chapter 26, "Weight Loss and Weight Control."

Percentage Body Fat

- Low body fat is common among elite athletes and is a goal of many aspiring competitors. However, no clear standards for body composition have been set for optimal performance in different sports.
- Various methods are available to assess body composition, the gold standard of which is hydrostatic weighing. See "Physical Tests" in Chapter 27, "History and Examination."

Diets

- Weight gain and weight loss programs should allow changes of no more than 2 lb/wk and should result in an improved lean to fat ratio of body composition.
- See Chapter 26, "Weight Loss and Weight Control."

CARBOHYDRATE

Carbohydrate should make up the majority of the athlete's diet. Athletes in heavy training must maintain a high intake of carbohydrate to sustain their activities.

Postexercise Repletion

- Daily repletion of glycogen reserves during training requires a dietary intake of up to 9 to 10 g of carbohydrate per kilogram of body weight, or 60% to 70% of total calories as carbohydrate, whichever is greater.
- Glycogen repletion should begin as soon as possible after exercise. About 0.7 g of carbohydrate per kilogram of body weight should be taken every 2 hours for the 4 to 6 hours after exercise.
- Simple sugars are more effective than starches and may be more acceptable after exercise in the form of liquid supplements.

Carbohydrate Loading

- Method #1: Reduce training efforts and increase carbohydrate intake during the 2 to 3 days just prior to competition. Body weight should increase by 1 to 2 kg.
- Method #2: Reduce carbohydrate intake to 50% of total calories for the first half of the week prior to competition while gradually reducing training intensity. During the second half of the week reduce training further while boosting carbohydrate intake to 70% of total calories or 10 g/kg of body weight.

Precompetition Meals

- Meals should be eaten 3 to 6 hours before the event.

- Meals should contain at least 100 g of carbohydrate and as much as 4.5 g/kg of body weight.
- Avoid carbohydrate 30 to 45 minutes prior to competition because of potential hypoglycemic reaction during the first few minutes of exercise.
- Carbohydrate intake within 30 minutes of the event is acceptable if it is easily digested.

Carbohydrate during Exercise

- Carbohydrate will improve performance if exercise lasts more than 1 hour.
- Liquid supplements may be more practical.
- Optimal range of intake appears to be 20 to 30 g of carbohydrate per half hour.
- Commercial sports drinks containing 6% to 8% carbohydrate as sucrose, glucose, fructose, and/or glucose polymer provide about 30 g of carbohydrate per 16 oz.
- Very intense exercise may benefit from higher concentrations (up to 25%) of glucose polymer solutions, but fluid replacement may not be optimal at these levels.

PROTEIN

- Protein requirements appear to be increased for many types of athlete.
- Intense training for any athlete may necessitate between 1.0 and 1.5 g of daily protein intake per kilogram of body weight.
- When training for muscle growth and increased strength, as much as 2 g/kg of body weight may be required for maximal protein retention.

- These amounts are commonly achieved with a normal 15% protein diet if calorie intake is large. Protein supplements therefore are not recommended.

FAT

- Fat intake must be limited in the athletic diet in order to accommodate the increased requirements for carbohydrate and protein.
- Dietary fat should represent less than 30% of the athlete's calorie intake.
- Saturated fat should be kept below 10% because of its association with many long-term health risks.

FLUID AND ELECTROLYTES

- Exercise, especially in high heat and/or humidity, causes significant losses of water, principally through sweating.
- Electrolyte losses are less significant; their replacement is necessary only during events lasting several hours.

Dehydration

Dehydration may deteriorate athletic performance and lead to hyperthermia.

Causes

- long, intense exercise sessions in warm, humid weather without adequate water intake
- voluntary restriction in wrestlers and other weight-class competitors

Prevention

- One to two cups of water 2 hours before training or competition and again 15 minutes before exercise should hydrate the tissues.
- During exercise, 4 to 8 oz of water every 10 to 15 minutes should be optimal, depending on exercise intensity and climate.
- Fluid losses should be monitored regularly by weighing the dry, nude body immediately before and after exercise.
- For each pound of body weight lost, 16 oz of fluid should be consumed within the next several hours.
- Weight loss over 2% of total body weight indicates that more fluids must be taken during exercise in the future.

Electrolyte Replacement

- Electrolyte replacement is necessary only for ultraendurance sports lasting over 4 hours.
- Most sports drinks supply acceptable amounts. Alternatively, the following recipe may be used: 1 qt of water + 1/2 cup of orange juice + 1/8 tsp of salt.

Water Intoxication or Hyponatremia

- Water intoxication is observed in ultraendurance athletes who are not accustomed to the heat and who drink low-sodium fluids, such as soft drinks, during competition.
- Sports drinks used in ultraendurance events should contain at least 230 mg of sodium, 195 mg of potassium, and 355 mg of chloride per quart.

VITAMINS

Deficiencies in Athletes

- It may be desirable for athletes to maximize vitamin intake within reasonable limits for the following reasons:
  1. Vitamins play essential roles in many aspects of cellular function during exercise.
  2. Exercise increases vitamin metabolism, which may increase requirements somewhat.
  3. Deficiencies of certain vitamins will produce measurable impairments of work performance.
- Most vitamins may be obtained in sufficient quantity from diet alone if the diet is well-balanced and contains enough calories. See Chapter 28, "Diet Analysis."

Supplements

- Limited information exists on the effects of vitamin supplementation on athletic performance.
- Some studies suggest that large daily doses of pantothenic acid (2000 mg) and vitamin C (1000 mg) are associated with positive performance effects.
- Some studies suggest that excesses of nicotinic acid (not niacinamide) and pyridoxine may impair performance.
- Vitamin E may be important in minimizing exercise-related damage to muscle tissue. Requirements may increase sufficiently to necessitate moderate supplemental intake. See "Vitamin E—Tocopherol" in Chapter 38, "Vitamins."

MINERALS

Deficiencies in Athletes

- Exercise may increase requirements for minerals such as magnesium, iron, zinc, and chromium.
- However, the increased food consumption associated with heavy training may minimize deficiency risks.

Supplements

- Mineral supplements have been shown to be of benefit in only two cases:
  1. "Phosphate-loading" with tribasic sodium phosphate, 4 g/d, produced measurable effects on endurance performance.
  2. Chromium, 200 µg/d as picolinate, has demonstrated an anabolic effect in weight lifters.

Calcium, Amenorrhea, and Bone Health

- Calcium intake is important in minimizing the effects of athletic amenorrhea on bone loss and stress fractures.
- Amenorrhea lasting 6 months or more must be evaluated and corrected to minimize risk of stress fracture.
- Reduction of training intensity and/or increased body weight may be necessary to restore normal menstrual cycle.

Iron and Anemia

- Iron deficiency is not uncommon among athletes and may cause impaired performance as well as poor health if not controlled.

- Clinical anemia may not be apparent, but serum ferritin levels below 20 µg/L indicate a problem.
- An athlete may have an "optimal" level of serum hemoglobin below which performance suffers, even if the level is within normal limits.
- Some athletes may demonstrate "pseudoanemia" due to exercise-induced increases in plasma volume. Treatment is not indicated.
- Athletes who are training heavily may regularly lose small quantities of blood due to hemolysis or bleeding from the gastrointestinal or genitourinary tracts.
- See Chapter 1, "Anemia."

ERGOGENIC AIDS

Many natural substances are promoted as ergogenic aids.

No Relevant Research

- Bee pollen, cytochromes, glandulars, royal jelly, spirulina, and succinate have not been subjected to controlled research on athletes.
- Medical research on branched-chain amino acids, and coenzyme Q_{10} has found uses for these substances in certain disease states only.

Positive Evidence

- Arginine and ornithine have not been shown to increase growth hormone levels in humans unless doses so large as to cause gastrointestinal side effects were employed.
- Preliminary human research suggests an anabolic effect for γ-oryzanol and ferulic acid (FRAC).

- Performance in anaerobic exercise may be enhanced by loading with bicarbonate or citrate. For example, sodium bicarbonate, 300 mg/kg of body weight, is taken in divided doses over 2.5 hours just prior to competition. Gastrointestinal side effects may occur.
- Endurance may be increased in some athletes by caffeine, 5 mg/kg of body weight prior to exercise, and carnitine, 2 to 6 g/d.
- One study reported that Chinese ginseng, 1000 mg/d, improved some aspects of endurance fitness and muscular strength.
- Tyrosine, 6 g/d, has been shown to have some positive effect on high-altitude physical and mental functioning.

Equivocal or Negative Evidence

- Conflicting research exists on the effects of octacosanol, 1000 µg/d, and mineral aspartates, 7 to 10 g/d.
- No beneficial effects have been found in controlled studies on inosine and pangamic acid (vitamin B15), also known as dimethylglycine (DMG).

26. Weight Loss and Weight Control

Any viable approach to weight loss must address calorie *consumption,* calorie *absorption* and/or calorie *expenditure.*

REDUCING CALORIE CONSUMPTION

An attempt should be made to assess the actual calorie needs of the individual.

Weight Maintenance Calorie Estimate

- 24 kcal/kg ideal weight for daily basal requirement
  +30% for sedentary activity
  +50% for light activity
  +75% for moderate activity
  +100% for heavy activity
- general formula—many exceptions may be encountered (see also Chapter 31, "Calories")

Diets

Mixed-Food Conventional Diet

- most logical choice for long-term compliance if patient's preferences can be accommodated

High-Protein/Fat, Low-Carbohydrate Diet

- higher satiety value
- side effects: reports of extreme fatigue, cardiac arrhythmias, hyperuricemia and gout, constipation, nausea, syncope, and calcium depletion
- may be dehydrating if sufficient water is not consumed
- linked with risk of atherosclerotic disease and some cancers

High Complex-Carbohydrate, Low-Fat Diet

- optimal diet for prevention of degenerative diseases
- extreme versions (Pritikin) have low satiety value and may cause compliance problems

Liquid Formula Diets

- popular with professionals and patients, but dismal long-term maintenance record
- care must be taken to provide all necessary nutrients, fiber, etc.

Very-Low-Calorie or Fasting Diets

These diets carry a high risk of complications:
- myocardial atrophy, congestive heart failure, glucose intolerance, hypotension, dehydration, ketoacidosis, sudden death
- weakness, irritability, nausea, edema, hair loss
- increased urinary excretion of potassium, calcium, magnesium, and nitrogen (from protein)
- increased blood levels of ketones, lactic acid, uric acid
- decreased blood levels of glucose, HDL cholesterol
- suppression of metabolic rate, which can become chronic if diets are used repeatedly

Diet Aids

Appetite Suppressants

- phenylethylamine derivatives
- only effective short-term, increasing tolerance requires larger doses
- all have major side effects, even nonprescription phenylpropanolamine, which can induce hypertension

Fiber Supplements

- not very effective, as satiety is short-lived and flatulence is a side effect
- may be necessary with liquid formula diets to ensure normal bowel function

Micronutrient Supplements

- indicated on low-calorie diets to guard against insufficient intake of essential vitamins and minerals

Support Groups

- Weight-Watchers, TOPS, Diet Workshop, Overeaters Anonymous
- very effective in encouraging compliance

Behavior Modification

- useful for changing poor eating habits without risk of physical side effects
- contingency contracting—achieving long-term goal wins prize
- positive reinforcement—frequent non-food rewards for abstaining

- stimulus control/environmental management—careful shopping, designated eating area, small plates, slow eating, removing temptations
- assertiveness training—learning to refuse food gracefully

Medical Procedures

- stomach bubble—has produced serious side effects

Surgery

- for life-threatening morbid obesity only
- gastroplasty (stomach stapling) only temporarily reduces food intake, has risk of complications

REDUCING CALORIE ABSORPTION

High-Fiber Diet

- no proof of any significant effect on absorption

Digestion Inhibitors (Starch Blockers)

- proven ineffective and potentially dangerous
- side-effects: nausea, vomiting, diarrhea, flatulence, and abdominal pain

Fat Substitutes

- sucrose polymers and other nonabsorbable compounds
- experimental, although approval of those proven safe is inevitable

Surgery

- for life-threatening morbid obesity only
- surgery examples: intestinal bypass, gastric bypass
- usually creates malabsorption syndromes

INCREASING CALORIE CATABOLISM

Human Chorionic Gonadotropin

- ineffective
- usually accompanied by 500 kcal diet

Thyroid Hormone

- stimulation of protein loss as well as fat
- side effect of increased myocardial irritability

Growth Hormone Stimulants

- arginine and ornithine
- trivial effect in animal studies only

Exercise

Aerobic Exercise

- Increases energy output depending on intensity and duration.
- Prolongs increase in metabolic rate (some studies).
- Helps appetite regulation.

- Encourages muscle sparing.
- Elevates mood.

Anaerobic Exercise

- Increases energy output depending on intensity and duration.
- May enhance metabolic rate by increasing amount of actively metabolizing tissue.
- See Chapter 25, "Sports Nutrition," for specific calorie costs of various types of exercise.

Bibliography for Part I: Clinical Protocols

General

Alpers DH, Clouse RE, Stenson WF. *Manual of Nutrition Therapeutics*. 2nd ed. Boston: Little, Brown and Co; 1988.

Austin S. *Clinical Nutrition* (seminars with bibliographies). Portland, Ore: Western States Chiropractic College; 1990–1991.

Austin S. *Clinical Nutrition Update* (periodical). Portland, Ore: Bergner Communications.

Bland JS. *Metabolic Update* (audio periodical with biblographies). Gig Harbor, Wash: HealthComm Inc; 1982–1985.

Bland JS. *Nutraerobics*. New York: Harper & Row; 1983.

Brown ML, ed. *Present Knowledge in Nutrition*. 6th ed. Washington, DC: International Life Sciences Institute-Nutrition Foundation; 1990.

Bouchard C, Shepard RJ, Stephens T, Sutton JR, McPherson BD, eds. *Exercise, Fitness and Health: A Consensus of Current Knowledge*. Champaign, Ill: Human Kinetics Publishers; 1988.

Buist R, ed. *International Clinical Nutrition Review* (periodical). Sydney, Australia: Integrated Therapies Pty, Ltd.

Committee on Diet and Health, Food and Nutrition Board, National Research Council, National Academy of Sciences. *Diet and Health: Implications for Reducing Chronic Disease Risk*. Washington, DC: National Academy Press; 1989.

Ensminger AH, Ensminger ME, Konlande JE, Robson JRK. *Foods and Nutrition Encyclopedia*. Clovis, Calif: Pegus Press; 1983.

Gaby AR, Wright JV. *Nutrition Therapy in Medical Practice* (seminar with bibliography). Los Angeles: Wright/Gaby Nutritional Seminars; 1985.

Halpern S. *Quick Reference to Clinical Nutrition*. 2nd ed. Philadelphia: JB Lippincott Co; 1987.

Hendler SS. *The Doctors' Vitamin and Mineral Encyclopedia*. New York: Simon and Schuster; 1990.

Krause MV, Mahan LK. *Food, Nutrition and Diet Therapy*. 7th ed. Philadelphia: WB Saunders Co; 1984.

Langseth L, ed. *Nutrition Research Newsletter* (periodical). Palisades, NY: Lyda Associates Inc.

Mckee G, ed. *Nutrition and the MD* (periodical). Los Angeles: PM Inc.

Monsen ER, ed. *Journal of the American Dietetic Association* (periodical). Chicago: American Dietetic Association.

Morgan BLG. *Nutrition Prescription: Strategies for Preventing and Treating 50 Common Diseases.* New York: Fawcett Crest; 1987.

Paige DM, ed. *Manual of Clinical Nutrition.* Pleasantville, NJ: Nutrition Publications Inc; 1983.

Pemberton CM, Moxness KE, German MJ, Nelson JK, Gastineau CF. *Mayo Clinic Diet Manual.* 6th ed. Philadelphia: BC Decker; 1988.

Pizzorno JE, Murray MT, eds. *A Textbook of Natural Medicine.* Seattle, Wash: John Bastyr College Publications; 1985.

Powers DE, Moore AO. *Food-Medication Interactions.* 6th ed. Tempe, AZ: F-M-I Publishers; 1988.

Shils ME, Young VR, eds. *Modern Nutrition in Health and Disease.* Philadelphia: Lea & Febiger; 1988.

US Department of Health and Human Services. *The Surgeon General's Report on Nutrition and Health: Summary and Conclusions.* Washington, DC: US Government Printing Office; 1988.

Werbach MR. *Nutritional Influences on Illness: A Sourcebook of Clinical Research.* Tarzana, Calif: Third Line Press; 1988.

Werbach MR. *Nutritional Influences on Mental Illness: A Sourcebook of Clinical Research.* Tarzana, Calif: Third Line Press; 1991.

Williams SR. *Nutrition and Diet Therapy.* St. Louis, Mo: CV Mosby Co; 1989.

Anemia

Bick RL, Baker WF. Iron deficiency anemia. *Lab Med.* 1990;21:641-648.

Chernoff R, ed. *Geriatric Nutrition: The Health Professional's Handbook.* Gaithersburg, Md: Aspen Publishers Inc; 1991.

Scates S, Glaspy J. The macrocytic anemias. *Lab Med.* 1990;21:736-741.

Arthritis

van de Laar MA, van der Korst JK. Rheumatoid arthritis, food, and allergy. *Semin Arthritis Rheum.* 1991;21:12-23.

Atherosclerosis and Cardiovascular Disorders

Hutchinson RG. *Coronary Prevention: A Clinical Guide.* Chicago: Year Book Medical Publishers; 1985.

Kritchevsky D. Antioxidant vitamins in the prevention of cardiovascular disease. *Nutr Today*. 1992;27:30-33.

Cancer

Ames BN. Dietary carcinogens and anticarcinogens. *Science*. 1983;221:1256-1264.

Committee on Diet, Nutrition, and Cancer, National Research Council. *Diet, Nutrition and Cancer*. Washington, DC: National Academy of Sciences; 1982.

Rensberger B. Cancer, the new synthesis: cause. *Science 84*. 1984;5:28-33.

Diabetes Mellitus

Anderson JW. *Nutrition Management of Metabolic Conditions*. Louisville, Ky: HCF Diabetes Research Foundation; 1988.

Powers MA, ed. *Nutrition Guide for Professionals*. Chicago: American Diabetes Association and American Dietetic Association; 1988.

Ravel R. *Clinical Laboratory Medicine: Clinical Application of Laboratory Data*. 5th ed. Chicago: Year Book Medical Publishers; 1989.

Food Allergy and Food Intolerance

Breneman JC. *Basics of Food Allergy*. 2nd ed. Springfield, Ill: Charles C Thomas; 1984.

Butkus SN, Mahan LK. Food allergy: immunological reactions to food. *J Am Diet Assoc*. 1986;86:601-608.

Rowe AH. *Food Allergy: Its Manifestations and Control and the Elimination Diets—A Compendium*. Springfield, Ill: Charles C Thomas; 1972.

Perkin J. *Food Allergies and Adverse Reactions*. Gaithersburg, Md: Aspen Publishers Inc; 1990.

Geriatric Nutrition

Chernoff R, ed. *Geriatric Nutrition: The Health Professional's Handbook*. Gaithersburg, Md: Aspen Publishers Inc; 1991.

Roe DA. *Geriatric Nutrition*. 3rd ed. Englewood Cliffs, NJ: Prentice Hall; 1991.

Simko MD, Cowell C, Hreha MS, eds. *Practical Nutrition: A Quick Reference for the Health Care Practitioner*. Gaithersburg, Md: Aspen Publishers Inc; 1989.

Gynecologic Disorders and Premenstrual Syndrome

Abraham GE. Nutritional factors in the etiology of the premenstrual tension syndromes. *J Reprod Med*. 1983;28:446-464.

Dawood MY, ed. *Dysmenorrhea*. Baltimore, Md: Williams & Wilkins Co; 1981.

Hypercholesterolemia and Related Lipid Disorders

National Cholesterol Educational Program. *Report of the Expert Panel on Detection, Evaluation and Treatment of High Blood Cholesterol in Adults.* Bethesda, Md: National Institutes of Health; 1988.

Hypertension

National High Blood Pressure Education Program. *The 1988 Report of the Joint Committee on Detection, Evaluation and Treatment of High Blood Pressure.* Bethesda, Md: National Institutes of Health; 1988.

Hypoglycemia and Related Disorders

Anderson JW. *Nutrition Management of Metabolic Conditions.* Louisville, Ky: HCF Diabetes Research Foundation; 1988.

Ravel R. *Clinical Laboratory Medicine: Clinical Application of Laboratory Data.* 5th ed. Chicago: Year Book Medical Publishers; 1989.

Watts NB, Keffer JH. *Practical Endocrinology.* 4th ed. Philadelphia: Lea & Febiger; 1989.

Immunity

Chandra RK, ed. *Nutrition and Immunology.* New York: Alan R Liss; 1988.

Van Buren C, Bach F, co-chairs. Symposium: update on immunonutrition. *Nutrition.* 1990;6(1):1-106.

Wan JMF, Haw MP, Blackburn GL. Nutrition, immune function and inflammation: an overview. *Proc Nutr Soc.* 1989;48:315-335.

Indigestion and Gastrointestinal Diseases

Floch MH. *Nutrition and Diet Therapy in Gastrointestinal Disease.* New York: Plenum Medical Book Co; 1981.

Fuller R. Probiotics in human medicine. *Gut.* 1991;32:439-442.

Shahani KM, Ayebo AD. Role of dietary lactobacilli in gastrointestinal microecology. *Am J Clin Nutr.* 1980;33:2448-2457.

Migraine Headache

Perkin JE, Hartje J. Diet and migraine: a review of the literature. *J Am Diet Assoc.* 1983;83:459-463.

Theisler C. *Migraine Headache.* Gaithersburg, Md: Aspen Publishers Inc; 1990.

Muscle Cramps

Gerber JM. Sports nutrition. In: Hazel R, Hyde T, eds. *Conservative Management of Sports Injuries.* Baltimore: Williams & Wilkins Co; in press.

Musculoskeletal Trauma

Gerber JM. Sports nutrition. In: Hazel R, Hyde T, eds. *Conservative Management of Sports Injuries.* Baltimore: Williams & Wilkins Co; in press.

Rayner H, Allen SL, Braverman ER. Nutrition in wound healing. *J Orthomol Med.* 1991;6:31-44.

Obesity, Weight Loss, and Weight Control

Frankle RT, Yang MU. *Obesity and Weight Control.* Gaithersburg, Md: Aspen Publishers Inc; 1988.

Katch FI, McArdle WD. *Nutrition, Weight Control, and Exercise.* 2nd ed. Philadelphia: Lea & Febiger; 1983.

Osteoporosis

Albanese AA. *Bone Loss: Causes, Detection and Therapy.* New York: Alan R Liss; 1977.

Chernoff R, ed. *Geriatric Nutrition: The Health Professional's Handbook.* Gaithersburg, Md: Aspen Publishers Inc; 1991.

Christiansen C, ed. Proceedings of a symposium: consensus development conference on osteoporosis. *Am J Med.* 1991;91(suppl 5B):1S-68S.

Pregnancy, Lactation, and Infancy

Committee on Nutrition, American Academy of Pediatrics. *Pediatric Nutrition Handbook.* Elk Grove Village, Ill: American Academy of Pediatrics; 1985.

Food and Nutrition Board, National Research Council. *Nutrition during Pregnancy.* Washington, DC: National Academy of Sciences; 1990.

Pipes PL. *Nutrition in Infancy and Childhood.* 4th ed. St. Louis, Mo: CV Mosby Co; 1989.

Simko MD, Cowell C, Hreha MS, eds. *Practical Nutrition: A Quick Reference for the Health Care Practitioner.* Gaithersburg, Md: Aspen Publishers Inc; 1989.

Worthington-Roberts BS. *Nutrition in Pregnancy and Lactation.* 4th ed. St. Louis, Mo: CV Mosby Co; 1989.

Zeiger RS. Prevention of food allergy in infancy. *Ann Allergy.* 1990;65:430-441.

Sports Nutrition

Burke LM, Read RSD. Sports nutrition: approaching the nineties. *Sports Med.* 1989;8:80-100.

Gerber JM. Sports nutrition. In: Hazel R, Hyde T, eds. *Conservative Management of Sports Injuries.* Baltimore: Williams & Wilkins Co; in press.

Grandjean AC, Storlie J, eds. *The Theory and Practice of Athletic Nutrition: Bridging the Gap, Report of the Ross Symposium.* Columbus, Ohio: Ross Laboratories; 1989.

Hickson JF, Wolinsky I, eds. *Nutrition in Exercise and Sport.* Boca Raton, Fla: CRC Press; 1989.

Lamb DR, ed. *Sports Science Exchange* (periodical). Chicago: Gatorade Sports Science Institute, Quaker Oats Co.

Part II
Clinical Assessment

27. History and Examination

CLINICAL APPROACH

Current Health Problems

- Assessment requires an adequate diagnostic evaluation in order to understand the condition affecting the patient.
- Assessment should result in a comprehensive treatment plan tailored to the patient's individual needs.
- Assessment should result in a strategy for implementation of a treatment plan that addresses issues of compliance, possible side effects, etc.
- Case management may require cotreatment with other professionals and an understanding of treatment interactions.

Preventive Health Care

- Assessment requires risk factor assessment utilizing many aspects of patient and family history, diet analysis, physical and laboratory evaluation.
- Assessment should result in prioritization of risks based on potential impact on future health in order to focus intervention effectively.
- Assessment should result in an individualized intervention plan with a strategy for implementation (see above).

PATIENT HISTORY

Personal Health History

- This portion of the history includes current and past complaints, medical and other treatments, and a review of systems.
- Comprehensive, self-administered questionnaires save the clinician's time while providing diagnostic clues. They also require the clinician to take responsibility for follow-up of new or worsening conditions.
- Beware of simplistic diagnostic systems using only signs and symptoms questionnaires. Most signs and symptoms suggest a variety of diagnoses, including non-nutritional ones.

Family History

- Family history is essential for risk factor assessment and preventive care.
- The history should include as many close blood relations as possible—siblings, parents, grandparents, aunts, uncles, etc. Ethnic background may also indicate specific risks.
- Family history may be obtained by questionnaire.

Environmental History

- Environmental history attempts to determine how the nutritional health of the individual is helped or hindered by aspects of the individual's life situation:
  1. socioeconomic level
  2. educational level
  3. occupation
  4. work/school/home environment

5. cultural beliefs and habits
6. family influences
7. disabilities
- Environmental history may be obtained by questionnaire.

Diet History

Many formats exist, all with their particular advantages and disadvantages. It is notoriously difficult to obtain information that is complete, detailed, and accurate.

Dietary Recall Interview

- The dietary recall interview attempts to elicit (1) "typical" intake (ie, usual breakfasts, lunches, dinners, snacks) or (2) intake over a recent specific time period (eg, most recent 24 hours).
  1. "Typical" recalls often give useful overviews of dietary habits but cannot be used for detailed nutrient analysis.
  2. Specific recalls gathered by trained interviewers can be accurate but are time-consuming and not necessarily typical of usual intake.

Food Diary

- The patient is asked to record intake over an extended period of time (eg, 7 days).
- Food diaries are practical for scanning the diet for certain problems (excess fat intake, low calcium intake).
- Food diaries are subject to falsification and may influence food choices. Accuracy depends on diligent recording of entire food, condiment, and beverage intake as well as portion sizes.
- In-depth analysis requires expert knowledge of foods or use of a computer program (see below).

Food Frequency Assessment

- The patient is asked to indicate the most common foods in his or her diet, specifying serving sizes and frequency per day, week, or month.
- Food frequency assessment may be done by using lists of foods that may be comprehensive or tailored to specific areas of concern (eg, dietary fat and cholesterol, fiber, iron, etc.).
- Food frequency assessment can be adapted for analysis by computer (see below).
- Comprehensive checklists are long and detailed; completing them can be tedious for the patient. Estimating frequency of consumption may be difficult for many patients.

Computerized Diet Analysis

- In-office program or outside vendor provides analysis of nutrient intake obtained from any of the above techniques.
- Clinician need not be involved in data collection or analysis if electronically scored frequency questionnaire is used. Detailed quantitative assessment of nutrient intake is possible.
- Results are only as good as patient input and available food data bases allow. Data entry may be time-consuming as well.

PHYSICAL TESTS

- Few nutrition-specific tests exist that are not part of general diagnostic examinations. Many physical signs of nutritional disease are not apparent until the condition is quite advanced.
- See individual entries for diagnostic evaluation in Part I: *Clinical Protocols.* See also entries for individual nutrients under "Deficiency Consequences" in Part III: *Macronutrients* and Part IV: *Micronutrients.*

- Muscle testing (kinesiology), although an attractive concept for easy diagnosis, has been shown to be ineffective for nutrition assessment in three different controlled studies.

Anthropometry

Anthropometry (body measurement) gives information about body composition and general health status.

Height and Weight

- Measurement requires a calibrated beam balance (not spring-loaded) scale.
- See Chapter 31, "Calories," and Appendix I for interpretive guidelines.

Wrist Circumference and Elbow Breadth

- Used to assess frame size which allows greater accuracy in evaluating body weight with standard height and weight tables.
- May give information on risk to age-related bone loss. See Chapter 22, "Osteoporosis."
- Wrist circumference method: Measure just distal to styloid processes on dominant arm. Divide height in centimeters by wrist circumference in centimeters and compare with the following values to obtain frame size estimate.

> Men: over 10.4 = small; under 9.6 = large.
> Women: over 11.0 = small; under 10.1 = large.
> Values between these extremes indicate medium frame.

- Elbow breadth method: See Table I-2 in Appendix I.

Body Fat Determinations

Skinfold Calipers

- Skinfold calipers are used to measure local subcutaneous fat thicknesses. These may be correlated with known standards or used in calculations for total body fat percentage.
- Caliper measurements are reliable in the hands of experienced and practiced users only. Infrequent use results in excessive operator errors.

Hydrostatic (Underwater) Weighing

- Hydrostatic weighing compares body weight in the air and during total submersion in water.
- This is very reliable and is the standard method by which other methods are evaluated; requires bulky and cumbersome equipment.

Bioelectric Impedance Analysis

- Bioelectric impedance analysis (BIA) is a relatively recent technology that uses a very low intensity electrical current to measure the electrical resistance of body tissues.
- Percentage fat values are falsely increased in dehydrated patients. BIA also is less accurate in subjects at upper and lower extremes of body fatness as well as after recent weight loss.

Ultrasound Measurement

- Ultrasound measurement has been investigated as an alternative to skinfold calipers in measuring local subcutaneous body fat.
- Thigh and biceps sites appear to best indicate overall body fatness. Accuracy is superior to calipers only in obese persons. Precision of portable units has not been examined.

Clinical Assessment 175

Infrared Interactance

- Infrared interactance also is being investigated as an alternative to skinfold calipers in measuring local subcutaneous body fat. Precision of portable units has not been examined.

Total-Body Electrical Conductivity, Neutron Activation, Magnetic Resonance, Isotope Dilution

- These techniques are used primarily in clinical research. Their potential usefulness in outpatient assessment is limited by cost and/or invasiveness.

Waist/Hip Ratio (Ponderosity Index)

- Used to identify fat distribution patterns, which more accurately reflect health risks.
- Method: Waist circumference is the smallest circumference measurement below the rib cage and above the umbilicus. Hip circumference is the largest circumference in the region of the buttocks.
- Ratios over 0.95 are associated with increasing risk of obesity-related disease. See Chapter 21, "Obesity."

Muscle Mass Determinations

Arm Muscle Circumference and Arm Muscle Area

- These are standard assessment tools for measuring body protein stores and detecting protein-calorie malnutrition.

Midarm Circumference and Triceps Skinfold Measurements

- Used in standard formulas or nomograms to calculate muscle dimensions.

Bone Densitometry

- Plain radiography is an insensitive and unreliable measure of bone density, especially in the spine and hip.
- Densitometry measurements of computed tomography (CT) images of spinal trabecular bone are sensitive but require considerable x-ray doses.
- Dual-photon absorptiometry is increasingly regarded as the tool of choice in bone mass assessment. Instruments are available for analyzing the radius, spine, or femoral neck.
- See Chapter 22, "Osteoporosis."

LABORATORY TESTS

- Laboratory tests are more useful for risk assessment (eg, serum lipoproteins) than nutritional diagnosis.
- Beware of diagnostic systems using artificially narrowed normal ranges for standard tests.
- See entries for individual nutrients under "Clinical Measurement" in Part III: *Macronutrients* and Part IV: *Micronutrients*. See also individual conditions in Part I: *Clinical Protocols*.

28. Diet Analysis

ASSESSMENT OF DIETARY DEFICIENCIES AND EXCESSES

- Assess dietary excesses of calories, total and saturated fats, cholesterol, protein, alcohol, refined sugar, salt, and certain additives if indicated.
- Assess dietary deficiencies of protein, vitamins, minerals, and dietary fiber.

Calories

- Optimal calories are difficult to measure for individuals because there are so many variables. A more practical evaluation can be done by answering the following questions:
  1. Is the patient within the ideal body weight range according to standard height and weight tables?
  2. Has the patient been gaining or losing weight steadily for the past few months?
- If the answers to the above questions indicate that the patient is at his or her ideal weight or is approaching such a weight at a reasonable pace (1 to 2 lb of weight change per week), then the calorie intake may be considered acceptable.
- See also Chapter 31, "Calories."

Total and Saturated Fat and Cholesterol

- These substances have all been associated with various degenerative diseases, notably atherosclerosis and some cancers.
- "Dietary Fat and Cholesterol Score" in Chapter 35, "Lipids and Lipid Factors," will give an estimate of their combined dietary load.

Dietary Fiber

- When inspecting a patient's diet, an intake of 8 to 10 servings per day of significant fiber-containing foods (see Chapter 34, "Dietary Fiber") should approach optimal levels.
- Patients with high risk factors for colon disease, atherosclerotic disease, biliary disease, and breast cancer should consume at *least* this amount.

Refined Sugar

- Inspect the patient's diet record for significant refined sugar sources (see Chapter 33, "Carbohydrates").
- The known, well-established risks of excessive refined sugar intake are limited to dental caries, gum disease, obesity, and possibly blood sugar disorders in sensitive persons (see Chapter 33).
- Although many patients may tolerate up to two servings of sweets per day, those with high risk of the above conditions should probably consume much less.

Salt

- Inspect the patient's diet record for significant sources of salt (see "Sodium" in Chapter 39, "Minerals").

- High salt intake may increase risk to hypertension and aggravate premenstrual syndrome and other types of edema, although not all patients with these problems are salt-sensitive.
- A low-salt diet would have *no* high sodium foods and allow *no* use of salt at the table and only small amounts in cooking.

ASSESSMENT OF PROTEINS AND MICRONUTRIENTS

Calculation of nutrient content of patient's diets by hand is not time-efficient for most professionals. Computer programs for the same purpose may be useful yet suffer from the great difficulty of keeping up with the expansion of variety in the American diet as well as the great variability in recipes for the same items. There is no substitute for direct inspection of the recorded diet by a professional who can recognize the signs of an inadequate diet without time-consuming calculations.

The "Modified Basic Four Food Guide" (see Chapter 29) and the "Food Group Exchange System" (see Chapter 30) are two assessment tools that provide methodologic approaches to the detection of nutrient deficiencies. Of the two, the exchange system is more precise and thorough yet requires more time and experience to implement.

29. Modified Basic Four Food Guide

Food group guides have been used to help classify foods eaten into groups representing elements of a balanced, adequate diet. The following appears to be the most accurate guide to date for achieving 100% of the RDA for adult diets (not pregnant or lactating; see Appendix H). Serving sizes may be adjusted to match overall calorie needs.

Dairy Products, Two or Three Servings per Day

- Dairy products are excellent sources of protein, vitamin B12, calcium, and zinc.
- Low-fat sources are recommended.
- See *Lactose Intolerance* under "Simple Sugars" in Chapter 33, "Carbohydrates," and Chapter 7, "Food Allergy" if dairy products are not well tolerated.

Animal Proteins, Two Servings per Day

- Animal proteins are excellent sources of protein, vitamin B6, B12, iron, zinc, chromium, and selenium.
- Low-fat sources are recommended.

Plant Proteins, Two Servings per Day

- Plant proteins (legumes, nuts, seeds) are excellent sources of vitamin B6, folic acid, magnesium, iron, copper manganese, chromium, and dietary fiber.

Whole-Grain Products, Four or More Servings per Day

- Whole-grain products (not white flour, white rice, etc.) are excellent sources of vitamin B6, manganese, chromium, selenium, and dietary fiber.
- Refined grain products are missing many of the above nutrients.

Total Fruits and Vegetables, Four or More Servings per Day

Include the following special subcategories:

Dark-Green Vegetables, One or More Servings per Day

- includes broccoli, Brussels sprouts, dark lettuces and cabbages, spinach, dark leafy greens (collards, turnip greens, etc.)
- excellent sources of vitamins A, E, and C, calcium, magnesium, iron, manganese, chromium, and dietary fiber

Vitamin C Foods, One or More Servings per Day

- includes citrus fruits, tomatoes, peppers, melons, strawberries, dark green leafy vegetables
- Excellent sources of vitamin C, folic acid, and dietary fiber

Polyunsaturated Oils, One Serving per Day

- includes most non-tropical plant and fish oils
- excellent sources of vitamin E and essential fatty acids

Avoid rancid oils that have been heated or stored beyond a reasonable shelf life (see "Unnatural Dietary Fats" in Chapter 35, "Lipids and Lipid Factors").

Table 29-1 lists quantitatively the nutrient contributions of the above food groups.

Table 29-1 Nutrient Density in Food Groups: Food Groups Containing at Least 5% of Recommended Allowances

Nutrient	Dairy (Not Cream Products)	Animal Protein (Flesh and Egg Dishes)	Vegetable Protein (Legumes, Nuts, and Seeds)	Whole-Grain (Not White Flour or Rice)	Vitamin C Vegetables/ Fruits	Dark Green Vegetable	Other Vegetables or Fruit	Oil (Vegetable Sources Only)
Protein	14–20%	25–50%	8–16%					
Vitamin A					20–40% (yellow noncitrus, tomato)	40–100%	20–100% (yellow-red vegetables)	
Vitamin E						20–25%		20–30%
Vitamin C					25–100%	25–100%	25–30% (cabbage)	
Vitamin B6		13–18% (not eggs)	13–18%	2–20%	10% (tomato)	5%	20% (banana) 9% (potato)	
Folic acid		12% (eggs)	12–36% (legumes)	10%	12–36%	12%	17% (beets)	
Vitamin B12	8–17%	17–33%						
Calcium	10–30%		5–15%			7–15%		
Magnesium	7% (not cheese)	7%	14% (not seeds)	7%		7–21%	14% (eggplant)	
Iron		6–17%	11%	6%		11%	28% (prunes)	
Zinc	7–13%	7–20%	3–7%	3–7%				
Copper		3–5%	10–15%	3–5%		3–5%	3–5%	
Manganese			10% (legumes) 30% (nuts)	10–30%		10%	5%	
Chromium	10–15% (cheese)	10–30%	20–30%	10%		10–15%	10–15%	
Selenium	15–25% (cheese)	25–60%		10–15%				

Note: Items in parentheses are the *only* examples in the category containing the indicated nutrient amounts.

30. Food Group Exchange System

BASIC PRINCIPLES AND RESOURCES

A very useful method for evaluating as well as designing diets is the food exchange system, originally developed for treating diabetes. In this system, the diet is broken down into categories of foods, such as dairy, meat, grain products, fruits, and vegetables. Each category has many members or exchanges, all of which contain similar amounts of calories and nutrients.

Exhibit 30-1 is an exchange category reference providing the following information:

- an extensive list of foods belonging to each exchange category, along with portion sizes
- lists of snacks and desserts, condiments, and beverages containing additional fat exchanges and added sugars
- a list of combination foods that contain more than one exchange category value
- a list of fiber exchanges

Table 30-1 depicts an exchange system suitable for evaluating and prescribing diets for most adults. The diet is divided into six categories of food:

- starches/bread
- lean to medium-fat proteins
- vegetables
- fruit
- milk products
- fats

Recommended servings are provided for various calorie intakes.

DIET ANALYSIS USING THE EXCHANGE SYSTEM

For diet analysis, food records are inspected and each food item is counted in terms of its exchange value(s) as well as the presence of added sugar and fiber. Exhibit 30-2 is a work sheet suitable for tallying exchange values, added sugar, and fiber.

Many meals contain multiple exchanges of one food. For example, a typical hamburger contains 4 oz of meat (four protein exchanges) on one bun (two starch/bread exchanges). A mixed dish, such as pizza, is composed of starch, protein, and fat exchanges (see Exhibit 30-1).

Total daily calories, carbohydrates, proteins, fats, added sugar, and fiber may be determined using the values for each exchange category. Percentage of total calories for carbohydrates, fats, and protein may be obtained from the following formulas:

% Carbohydrate = [(grams carbohydrate $\times$ 4)/(total calories)] $\times$ 100%
% Protein = [(grams protein $\times$ 4)/(total calories)] $\times$ 100%
% Fat = [(grams fat $\times$ 9)/(total calories)] $\times$ 100%

Micronutrient balance may be estimated by referring to Table 30-1. If the minimal numbers of servings for each category are present for the calorie level consumed, the diet may be considered adequate.

DIET PRESCRIPTION USING THE EXCHANGE SYSTEM

In prescribing a diet, instruct the patient to eat daily a predetermined number of servings from each category: starch/bread, proteins, vegetables, fruit, milk products, and fats. The goal is to achieve the intake of the desired amount of calories, carbohydrates, protein, fat, and micronutrients. The patient is free to make choices within each allowed category.

To prescribe a diet, first determine the desired calorie intake. This may be done by analyzing the patient's current diet or by using calculations explained elsewhere. See Chapter 25, "Sports Nutrition," and Chapter 31, "Calories." When the desired calorie level is known, Table 30-1 may be consulted for the ideal number of exchanges from each food category that should be included in the daily diet. Four typical calorie intakes (plus two meatless plans) are shown and extrapolations may be made to accommodate other calorie levels.

Familiarity with the portion sizes of exchange items is key to the successful application of this system. Patient education tools may be obtained from either the American Diabetes Association or the American Dietetic Association. This exchange system provides a high-carbohydrate, moderate-protein, low-fat diet with fairly adequate vitamin and mineral balance. However, such plans have been shown to be often insufficient in micronutrient levels. Therefore, additional recommendations for maximizing micronutrient intakes have also been supplied (see Choices To Emphasize for Maximal Daily Micronutrients in Table 30-1).

Within exchange categories, certain micronutrients may be emphasized when necessary as in the following examples:

- Carotene intake may be increased with yellow-red fruits and vegetables from the *fruit* and *vegetables* categories.
- Calcium intake may be increased by including more cheese choices from the *protein* category.
- Iron intake may be increased by using red meats from the *protein* category as well as fortified breakfast cereals and legumes from the starch/bread category.

Exhibit 30-1 Food Choices in Exchange System Categories

Note: When the item is followed by superscripts (eg, granola$^{(1,0)}$), the first number indicates additional fat exchanges and the second number indicates added sugar exchanges. These will increase total calorie, carbohydrate, and/or fat intakes. Key: C = carbohydrate; P = protein; F = fat; g = grams; tr = trace.

Starches/bread (80 kcal, 15g C, 3g P, tr F)
3 Tbs Grape-Nuts, wheat germ; 1/3 cup All-Bran, Bran-Buds
1/2 cup bran flakes, shredded wheat, cooked cereals, grits
3/4 cup unsweetened breakfast cereals, 1 1/2 cups puffed cereal, 1/4 cup granola$^{(1,0)}$
1 oz low/moderate/high sugar breakfast cereal (1–3 added sugar exchanges)
1/3 cup cooked rice, 1/2 cup cooked pasta, Oriental noodles,$^{(1,0)}$ 1/3 cup bread stuffing$^{(1,0)}$
1 slice bread, 1/2 bagel, bun, English muffin, pita, 2 taco shells$^{(1,0)}$
1 small roll, tortilla, small biscuit,$^{(1,0)}$ 1 small plain muffin,$^{(1,0)}$ 1/2 large specialty muffin$^{(1,0)}$
2 small pancakes,$^{(1,0)}$ 1 small waffle,$^{(1,0)}$ 1 slice French toast$^{(1,0)}$
2-in cube corn bread,$^{(1,0)}$ 1 croissant/crescent roll$^{(2,0)}$
2 bread sticks, 1 cup low-fat croutons
3/4 oz low-fat crackers, pretzels, matzo, 3/4 oz (6–10) snack crackers$^{(1,0)}$
3 cups air-popped corn, oil-popped corn,$^{(1,0)}$ microwave or buttered popcorn$^{(2,0)}$
1 oz fried potato chips, corn chips, tortilla chips, etc.$^{(2,0)}$
1/2 cup corn, lima beans, green peas, plantain, mashed potato
1 small potato, 6-in corn on cob, 1 cup winter squash
1/3 cup yam, sweet potato, 10 (1.5 oz) French fries$^{(1,0)}$
1/2 cup hash-brown potatoes$^{(2,0)}$
2 oz (4 large) onion rings$^{(2,0)}$
1/4 cup baked beans; 1/3 cup cooked lentils, beans, peas, refried beans, hummus$^{(1,0)}$
1/2 cup bean salad$^{(0,1)}$

Lean protein (55 kcal, 0g C, 7g P, 3g F)
1 oz lean beef (round, sirloin, flank, tenderloin), wild game
1 oz ham, Canadian bacon, pork tenderloin, veal chops and roasts
1 oz skinless chicken, turkey, Cornish hen
1.5 oz very-low-fat (95%) luncheon meat
1 oz fresh or frozen fish, 6 oysters, 2 sardines
2 oz shellfish, 1/4 cup water-pack tuna
1/4 cup cottage cheese, 2 Tbs Parmesan cheese, 1 oz very-low-calorie diet cheeses
3 egg whites, 1/2 cup low-calorie egg substitutes
1/4 cup vegetarian burger, tempeh

Medium-fat protein (75 kcal, 0g C, 7g P, 5g F)
1 oz most beef products except prime cuts and corned beef
1 oz most pork products except ribs, ground pork, and sausage

(continues)

Exhibit 30-1 Continued

1 oz most lamb products except ground lamb
1 oz unbreaded veal cutlet, 1 oz low-fat (86%) luncheon meat
1 oz poultry with skin, duck or goose, ground turkey
1/4 cup canned salmon, oil-pack tuna
1 oz fried seafood or chicken
1 oz mozzarella, other part-skim cheeses, diet cheeses
1/4 cup ricotta cheese
1 egg, 1/4 cup egg substitutes
1 oz liver, other organ meats
1/2 cup soft tofu, 1/4 cup firm tofu, 1 cup soy milk

High-fat protein (100 kcal, 0g C, 7g P, 8g F) (may be counted as 1 medium-fat protein + 1 added fat exchange)
1 oz corned beef, prime rib, sausage, ribs, regular luncheon meat, 1 turkey/chicken frankfurter, 1 beef/pork frankfurter[(1,0)]
1 oz most cheeses
1 Tbs peanut butter, 1 oz peanuts/almonds/seeds[(1,0)]

Vegetables (25 kcal, 5g C, 2g P, 0g F)
1/2 cup cooked, 1 cup raw vegetables
1/2 cup tomato sauce, 1/2 cup spaghetti sauce(1,2)
See *starches/bread* category for starchy vegetables

Fruit (60 kcal, 15g C, 0g P, 0g F)
1 medium-size whole fruit
1/2 cup most fresh fruit, unsweetened canned fruit, or juice
1 cup most berries, grapes, papaya, melons

1/4 cup most dried fruit (less of sweeter types)
1/2 banana, grapefruit, mango, pomegranate
1/2 cup canned fruit in syrup,[(0,3)] 1/2 cup sweetened applesauce[(0,3)]

Milk products (90 kcal, 12g C, 8g P, tr F)
1 cup 0 to 1% fat milk, buttermilk, yogurt
1/3 cup nonfat dry milk powder, 1/2 cup evaporated skim milk
1 cup flavored nonfat yogurt[(0,5)]
1 cup nonfat frozen yogurt[(0,6)]
similar amounts of low-fat or whole-milk products (1–2 added fat exchanges per serving)
1 cup chocolate milk[(1,3)]
1 small milkshake[(2,10)]
1 cup milk pudding[(1,10)]
1 cup custard[(3,3)]

Fats (45 kcal, 5g F); equals one added fat exchange per serving
1 tsp butter, margarine, mayonnaise, vegetable oil
1 Tbs diet margarine, low-calorie mayonnaise, cream cheese
2 Tbs sour cream, 2 Tbs coffee creamer
2 tsp cheese salad dressing
1 Tbsp creamy/oil-type salad dressing, low-calorie cheese salad dressings
2 Tbs low-calorie oil-type salad dressing
1/4 cup rich sauces/gravies, 1/2 cup regular sauces/gravies
10 large/20 small peanuts, 4 halves walnuts, pecans
1 Tbs most seeds, cashews, other nuts; 2 tsp pumpkin seeds

(continues)

Exhibit 30-1 Continued

5 large/10 small olives, 1/8 avocado, 2 Tbs coconut
1 slice bacon, 1 sausage link, 1/2 ounce chitterlings

Snacks and desserts (added fat and sugar only)
1 small doughnut,[1,1] unfrosted brownie[1,1]
1 piece angel food cake,[0,4] 1 oz Animal Crackers,[0,4] fig/fruit Newtons[0,4]
1 piece fruitcake,[1,4] sponge cake,[1,4] cupcake[1,4]
1 small sweet roll[1,2]
2 oz most pastries/Danish[2,6]
1 piece most cakes,[2,4] 1 slice fruit pie,[2,5] 1 slice cream pie,[3,5] 1 fried snack pie[3,5]
1 slice cheesecake[3,6]
2–3 most small cookies,[1,3] 5–7 snap/wafer cookies[1,3]
1 fruit/pudding frozen confection[0,2]
1 small cone ice cream/frozen yogurt/soft serve[1,4]
1/2 cup premium frozen dessert and ice cream/bars/sandwiches[3,5]
1/2 cup sherbet/fruit ice[0,5]
1 fast-food ice cream sundae[2,10]
1/2 cup gelatin dessert[0,4]
1 oz toffee/jelly/hard candy[0,4]
1 small granola dessert bar[1,3]
1 oz most candy,[0,5] 1 oz most chocolate-coated bars[1,5]
1 oz all-chocolate candy,[1,3] 1 oz all-chocolate candy with nuts[2,3]
2 pieces chewing gum/1 piece bubble gum[0,1]

Sweet condiments (added fat and sugar only)
1 tsp sugar,[0,1] 1 Tbs molasses,[0,3] 2 Tbs cake frosting,[1,6] 1 Tbs honey,[0,4] 2 Tbs pancake syrup,[0,5] 2 Tbs chocolate syrup[0,6]
1 Tbs jam/jelly,[0,2] 1/3 cup sweetened coconut[2,2]
1 Tbs barbeque sauce or seasoning,[0,1] 1 Tbs sweet relish,[0,1] 2 Tbs catsup,[0,1] 1 small sweet pickle[0,2]

Beverages (added fat, sugar and/or calories only)
1 cup flavored coffee[0,1]
8 oz sports drink[0,3]
1 cup cocoa[0,4]
8 oz fruit-flavored drink[0,6]
12 oz soft drinks[0,10]
12 oz regular beer (150 kcal), 12 oz light beer (100 kcal)
3.5 oz wine (70 kcal), 12 oz wine cooler[0,7] (+100 kcal)
1.5 oz liqueurs/fruit brandy[0,5] (+100 kcal)
1.5 oz hard liquor (100 kcal)

Combination foods
Key: S = starch; LP = lean protein; MFP = medium-fat protein; HFP = high-fat protein; V = vegetable; D = milk product; F = added fat; AS = added sugar

1 cup casserole (2S, 2MFP, 1F)
8 oz pot pie (3S, 2MFP, 2F)
1 cup beef stew (1S, 2MFP), chicken stew (1S, 2LP)

(continues)

Exhibit 30-1 Continued

1 cup bean entree (2S, 1LP, 1F)
1 large slice cheese pizza (2S, 1MFP, 1F)
1 cup chili with beans (2S, 2MFP, 2F)
1 cup Oriental stir-fry (1V, 1LP, 1F)
1 cup macaroni and cheese (2S, 1MFP, 2F)
1 cup bean soup (1S, 1V, 1LP)
1 can chunky soup (1S, 1V, 1MFP)
1 cup cream soup (1S, 1F)
1 cup most pasta with meat (2S, 1MFP, 1F)
1 cup meat lasagna (2S, 2MFP)
1 jumbo fast-food hamburger (3S, 4MFP, 2F)
1 quarter-pounder hamburger (2S, 3MFP, 1F)
1 cheeseburger (2S, 2MFP, 1F)
1 regular hamburger (2S, 2MFP)
1 tuna salad sandwich (2S, 2MFP, 1F)
1 breakfast egg muffin (2S, 2MFP, 1F)
1 breakfast sausage muffin (2S, 2HFP, 2F)
1 two-egg omelette w/ham and cheese (2MFP, 1F)
1 cup whole-milk instant breakfast (1S, 1LP, 1D, 1F, 2AS)
1 large breakfast bar (1S, 1MFP, 1F, 1AS)
2–3 small diet bars (1S, 1MFP, 2F, 2AS)
1 can liquid diet meal (1S, 1D, 1F, 3AS)
1 taco (1S, 1MFP, 1F)
2 small meat/cheese enchiladas (2S, 2HFP)
1 meat burrito (3S, 2HFP)
1/2 cup coleslaw (1V, 1F, 1AS)
1/2 cup pasta salad (2S, 2F, 1AS)
1/2 cup potato salad (1S, 2F)
1/2 cup tuna salad (4LP, 4F)

Dietary fiber
May be estimated from the following exchange values:
 high-bran products—8 g/exchange
 moderate-bran products—4 g/exchange
 whole-grain products—2 g/exchange
 legumes—3 g/exchange
 starchy vegetables—3 g/exchange
 other vegetables—2 g/exchange
 berries—4 g/exchange
 most fruits, raisins, dates—2 g/exchange
 most dried fruit—4 g/exchange

Table 30-1 Food Exchange Plan for Optimal Health

Food Group	Exchanges per Day						Choices to Emphasize for Maximal Daily Micronutrients
	1200 kcal*	1500 kcal*	2000 kcal	2500 kcal	1400 kcal* Meatless	1900 kcal* Meatless	
Starches, bread, without fat	7	9	12	14	8	12	Use whole-grain products
Lean to medium-fat proteins	3	4	6	6	0	0	Include 2–4 servings legumes Use red meats and dark poultry meats
Vegetables	3	4	5	6	4	5	Include dark green and yellow/orange
Fruit	2	2	3	6	3	4	Include citrus and yellow/orange
Milk products, 1% fat or less	2	2	2	3	4	4	
Added fats	1	2	3	4	2	4	Include polyunsaturated
Approximate Nutrient Content As Percentage of Total Calories							
Carbohydrate (g)	58%	56%	55%	59%	66%	66%	
Protein (g)	21%	21%	21%	19%	18%	16%	
Fat (g)	21%	24%	25%	23%	17%	19%	

Note: Actual calorie levels are ±100 kcal. One added sugar exchange contains 16 kcal. Five added sugar exchanges (see Exhibit 30-1) replace the calories and carbohydrates but *not* vitamins and minerals in one starch exchange.

*Low-calorie diets and diets low in animal products may require vitamin/mineral supplementation.

Exhibit 30-2 Work Sheet for Diet Analysis Using Food Group Exchange System

Food Item	Portion Size	Starch/bread	Low-fat protein	Medium-fat protein	High-fat protein	Vegetables	Fruit	Milk product	Fat	Sugar	Fiber	GRAND TOTALS
	Total exchanges											
	Calories											
	Carbohydrate											
	Protein											
	Fat											

Bibliography for Part II: Clinical Assessment

American Diabetes Association and American Dietetic Association. *Exchange Lists for Meal Planning*. Chicago: American Dietetic Association; Alexandria, Va: American Diabetes Association; 1986.

King JC, Cohenour SH, Corrucini CG, Schneeman P. Evaluation and modification of the basic four food guide. *J Nutr Educ*. 1978;10:39-41.

Krause MV, Mahan LK. *Food, Nutrition and Diet Therapy*. 7th ed. Philadelphia: WB Saunders Co; 1984.

Pennington J. *Food Values of Portions Commonly Used*. 15th ed. New York: Harper & Row; 1989.

Powers MA, ed. *Nutrition Guide for Professionals*. Chicago: American Diabetes Association and American Dietetic Association; 1988.

Pressman AH, Adams AH. *Clinical Assessment of Nutritional Status: A Working Manual*. 2nd ed. Baltimore: Williams & Wilkins Co; 1990.

Roche AF, ed. *Body-Composition Assessments in Youth and Adults: Report of the Sixth Ross Conference on Medical Research*. Columbus, Ohio: Ross Laboratories; 1985.

Simko MD, Cowell C, Hreha MS, eds. *Practical Nutrition: A Quick Reference for the Health Care Practitioner*. Gaithersburg, Md: Aspen Publishers Inc; 1989.

Part III
Macronutrients

31. Calories

CALORIES AND NUTRITION

US Adult Intake

- men: 1200 to 5000 kcal/d range, 2500 average
- women: 700 to 3000 kcal/d range, 1500 average

Caloric Value of Nutrients

- lipids—9 kcal/g
- protein—4 kcal/g
- alcohol—7 kcal/g
- carbohydrates—4 kcal/g

Calorie-Dense Foods

- high-fat: 6-oz steak, 600 kcal; bacon, 50 kcal per slice; Big Mac, 560 kcal; ice cream, 130 to 200 kcal per scoop; French fries, 220 kcal per serving; cheese pizza, 160 kcal per slice; Kentucky Fried Chicken dinner, 700 kcal
- high-alcohol: beer, 100 to 150 kcal per can; wine, 75 to 150 kcal per glass; hard liquor, 75 kcal/oz
- high-sugar: soft drinks, 150 kcal per can; pie/cake, 200 to 400 kcal per piece; breakfast cereal, 110 kcal/oz; Milky Way, 260 kcal

Empty Calories

- Empty calories are calories added to foods without increasing other nutrients:
  1. high-fat meat produced by overfeeding livestock
  2. refined carbohydrates with reduced vitamin, mineral, and fiber content
  3. fried foods (fat absorbed during frying)
  4. table sugar, table fats, desserts, soft drinks, alcohol, etc.
- Average American diet has 36.8% of its calories as foods that are *not* in the basic food groups.
- Empty calories increase likelihood of micronutrient undernutrition.

CALORIE REQUIREMENTS

Estimated Average RDA for Ages 19 to 50 Years

- men—2900 kcal/d or 37 to 40 kcal/kg of body weight; women—2200 kcal/d or 36 to 38 kcal/kg of body weight
- variation among similar individuals with comparable activity levels possibly ± 40%
- influenced by three major factors: resting metabolic rate (RMR), diet-induced thermogenesis, and physical activity

Resting Metabolic Rate

- RMR is minimal energy needed at rest.
- RMR can vary as much as 30% between similar individuals.
- Low rates are found in individuals with (1) low proportion of lean body mass, (2) severely restrictive dieting habits, and (3) low levels of thyroid or adrenal hormones.

- RMR may be estimated roughly in adults by the following formulas: for women, $0.9 \times IBW \times 24$; for men, $1.0 \times IBW \times 24$, where IBW is ideal body weight in kilograms.

Diet-Induced Thermogenesis

- Diet-induced thermogenesis is increased heat production after a meal.
- Diet-induced thermogenesis increases calorie requirements 5 to 10% on average.
- It is caused in part by energy production needed to digest, absorb, and metabolize food.
- Some individuals may be genetically capable of adjusting the level of this response to the size of the meals they consume, minimizing weight fluctuations. They may feel uncomfortably warm after a large meal.

Physical Activity

- Intensity and duration of physical activity determines calorie requirement.
- The daily calorie requirement must be increased over resting levels, depending on average activity level (sedentary, very light, moderate, heavy) and special demands such as strenuous athletic training (see below).

Other Factors

- Factors that increase calorie requirements include: growth, larger body size, and extremes of environmental temperature.
- Factors that decrease requirements include: lower lean body mass and aging.

Estimating Total Energy Requirements

- A 24-hour day must be divided into hours spent at each of the following activity levels:
  1. resting—RMR × 1.0 × (hours/24)
  2. sedentary activity (driving, typing)—RMR × 1.5 × (hours/24)
  3. light activity (slow walk, light work)—RMR × 2.5 × (hours/24)
  4. moderate activity (load carrying, dancing)—RMR × 5.0 × (hours/24)
  5. heavy activity (heavy manual labor or exercise)—RMR × 7.0 × (hours/24)
- Adding the contributions of each category will provide the total daily calorie needs.

CLINICAL MEASUREMENT

Pediatric Growth Charts

- Changes in both length and weight from month to month are useful nutritional indices, but weight measurements are usually more accurate.
- Head circumference changes are not very useful.
- Extremely high or low percentile rankings may be significant, as may sharp deviations from previous percentile rankings.

Height and Weight Tables

- These tables were developed for assessing mortality risk, not optimal health. They were derived from insurance policyholders only, which may introduce bias.
- Most height and weight tables require measurement of frame size from wrist circumference or elbow breadth. See "Physical Tests" in Chapter 27, "History and Examination."

- Health risks of excess weight may begin above 110% of the mean for male-pattern fat distribution (mostly trunk fat), especially in younger adults and if other risk factors exist. Male-pattern fat distribution is defined as a waist/hip circumference ratio (ponderosity index) greater than 0.95 (see Chapter 27).
- Female-pattern fat distribution (mostly pelvic/thigh fat) may not be at risk until it surpasses 130%.
- Health risks of being underweight begin below 85% for males and females.

Body Mass Index

- Body mass index (BMI) is calculated by dividing weight by the square of height. Must use kilograms (divide pounds by 2.2) and meters (divide inches by 39.4).
- Health risks begin at BMI above 25 and are serious above 30.

Body Composition Analysis

- Body composition analysis (see Chapter 27, "History and Examination") is done by
  1. underwater weighing
  2. skinfold caliper measurement
  3. bioelectric impedance
  4. infrared interactance
  5. ultrasound analysis
- Body composition analysis attempts to isolate the fat compartment, which is most clinically important.
- Optimal levels have not been established. Acceptable ranges appear to be 13% to 18% for men and 22% to 28% for women. Different techniques may not produce same numerical results.

Metabolic Rate Factors

- Thyroid dysfunction: Clinical abnormalities are detectable by serum levels of thyroxine and thyroid-stimulating hormone.
- Basal body temperature: Axillary measurement below 97.5°F suggests low metabolic rate according to some authorities.

CALORIE IMBALANCES

Calorie Deficiency

- Calorie deficiency is uncommon in the United States except in extreme poverty, extreme malabsorption, certain degenerative conditions (cancer), and psychologic disorders (anorexia nervosa), and in certain weight-conscious athletes (wrestlers, boxers, swimmers, dancers, figure skaters, gymnasts, jockeys, etc.).
- Increases risk of death in chronic obstructive pulmonary disease and cancer.
- May contribute to amenorrhea in female athletes.
- Intake below 1800 kcal/d increases risk for micronutrient deficiencies.

Calorie Excess

- Obesity is defined as more than 20% above ideal body weight.
  1. total population—25% obese
  2. female population—35% obese
- Overweight is defined as 10% to 20% above ideal body weight.
  1. male population—18.1% overweight
  2. female population—12.6% overweight
- Obesity is associated with hypertension, hyperlipidemia, heart disease, diabetes, some cancers, gallbladder disease, gynecologic

disorders, osteoarthritis, gout, surgical complications, and social discrimination.
- Twenty-five percent of children are obese according to triceps skinfold measurements. This represents a large, recent increase in obesity in the pediatric population.

32. Alcohol

HEALTH HAZARDS

Excessive Intake Increases Risk of

- heart disease, hypertension, stroke, hypertriglyceridemia
- gastrointestinal and breast cancer
- cirrhosis of the liver, gastritis, pancreatitis, diabetes
- anemia, immune deficiency
- peripheral neuritis, central nervous system dysfunction
- fetal/neonatal abnormalities
- hypoglycemia via hormone imbalance, liver impairment or autonomic dysfunction
- impotence and lowered testosterone (male), early menopause (female)
- bone changes and skeletal deformities

Conditions That May Worsen with Moderate Intake

- Cardiac arrhythmia and cardiomyopathy

Effects on Nutrition

- Alcohol replaces nutritious food with empty calories, which increases vitamin B complex requirements.
- Alcohol irritates gastrointestinal mucosa and impairs organs of digestion, predisposing malabsorption, especially of thiamine and vitamins A, D, K, B6, B12, C, and folic acid.

- Alcohol impairs liver uptake and/or activation of vitamins D, B1, B6, and folic acid. It depresses metabolism of amino acids.
- Alcohol causes increased excretion of calcium, magnesium, and zinc.
- Alcohol metabolism results in an increase in oxygen free radicals, which may require increased nutritional support of antioxidant systems. This includes adequate intake of vitamin B complex, sulfur amino acids such as cysteine, vitamins C and E, and selenium and zinc.

HEALTH BENEFITS OF MODERATE INTAKE

- One to three drinks per day in healthy adult men and postmenopausal women may improve HDL levels and reduce risk of coronary and cerebral thrombosis.
- Moderate intake reduces incidence of gallstones.

SCREENING

Signs of Problem Drinking

- It adversely affects any of the following: home life, work, finances, reputation, ambition, sleep habits, personal efficiency, memory.
- It is used to deal with shyness, worries, lack of self-confidence.
- It results in guilt, undesirable associations, cravings for drink, drinking alone, medical treatment.

NUTRITION AND RECOVERY

- A nutritionally adequate diet is essential with supplements if deficiency has been severe.

- Treatment of existing hypoglycemia has been suggested to help control cravings.
- One study suggested that glutamine, 2 g/d, may help control cravings.
- Pantethine, a metabolite of vitamin B5, may reduce toxic effects of chronic alcohol consumption.

HANGOVER MANAGEMENT

- bland foods for gastrointestinal upset
- clear soups for water and electrolyte replacement
- fruit juices for low blood sugar
- caffeine beverages for vascular headache

33. Carbohydrates

SIMPLE SUGARS

Occurrence

- natural sources: lactose in milk; fructose, glucose and sucrose in fruits
- other sources: added table sugar, corn syrup, corn sweetener, invert sugar, brown sugar, honey, molasses, maple syrup
- high-sugar foods: cakes, cookies, pastries—up to 80 g per serving; ice cream desserts—up to 56 g per serving; soft drinks—40 g per serving; breakfast cereal—up to 15 g per serving; candy—up to 40 g per serving; jams and jellies—up to 40 g/oz; canned fruits in syrup—12 g per serving; flavored yogurt—20 g per serving

Food Sweeteners

- dextrose—glucose, 0.7 times sweeter than sucrose
- levulose—fructose, 1.7 times sweeter than sucrose
- raw sugar—96% sucrose, 4% molasses; cane sugar byproduct
- molasses—50% or less sucrose
- brown sugar—sucrose with added molasses
- sorghum syrup—sucrose extract of sorghum plant
- corn syrup—glucose from cornstarch
- corn sweetener—corn syrup partially (40% to 100%) converted to fructose
- invert sugar—50/50 mixture of glucose and fructose

- honey—50/50 mixture of glucose/fructose; tupelo has more fructose
- maple syrup—mostly sucrose

Intake

- US average is 24% of total calories (18% refined), previously 18% of total calories (12% refined) in 1900.
- Recommended intake (refined) is no more than 10% of total calories. Up to two servings of nonfruit sweets may be acceptable in low-risk individuals (see below).

Associated Health Risks

Dental Caries and Gum Disease

- Sugars are most hazardous when allowed to stick to teeth or remain in mouth for extended periods.

Sugar Intolerance

- Human studies utilizing extremely high sugar intakes over a short time have shown that blood sugar homeostasis is impaired by such intakes. No long-term studies using more realistic diets have been performed.
- Of US adults 9% to 17% have genetic tendency toward sugar intolerance and are likely to be more sensitive to the current US high-sugar diet.

Cardiovascular Disease

- Sugar contributes to high triglyceride levels and early atherosclerosis in sugar-sensitive adults only.

Cancer

- Preliminary studies suggest a weak association of sugar with breast cancer.

Lactose Intolerance

- Lactose intolerance is found in some infants and many non-Caucasian adults who react to milk ingestion with bloating, cramps, and diarrhea.
- Ninety percent of Asians, 70% of African Americans, 65% of Hispanics, and only 15% of Caucasians lose sufficient lactase activity in adulthood to become lactose-intolerant.
- Condition is verified by challenge with 16 oz of milk, lactose intolerance test, or hydrogen breath test.
- Lactose-reduced milk, lactase milk enzyme, or lactase digestive aids are available over-the-counter for intolerant individuals. Yogurt and some cheeses may be well tolerated.

Sugar Substitutes

- saccharin—synthetic, suspected carcinogen
- cyclamate—synthetic, suspected carcinogen
- aspartame—synthetic, health risks controversial (Some critics fear large amounts may cause neurologic damage to fetuses and children. Some adults may be sensitive and react with headache, rashes, or neurologic symptoms.)
- acesulfame-K—synthetic, undergoing safety testing prior to approval
- mannitol, sorbitol—natural, nutritive, noncariogenic, possible diarrhea in large amounts
- xylitol—natural, nutritive, noncariogenic, possible diarrhea, possible carcinogen

Note: Despite the popularity of non-nutritive sweeteners, the average intake of sugar and the average weight of Americans remain *unchanged.*

COMPLEX CARBOHYDRATES (STARCHES)

Occurrence

- grains and grain products—wheat, corn, rice, oats, barley, millet, rye, buckwheat, triticale, amaranth (Products include breads and other baked goods, breakfast cereals, pastas, popcorn, and other snacks.)
- nuts—10% to 27% carbohydrate
- legumes (seed vegetables)—peanuts, beans, peas, lentils
- root/tuber vegetables—potatoes, yams, carrots, rutabagas, water chestnuts
- gourd vegetables—winter squashes (acorn, hubbard, etc.), pumpkin
- modified food starch—additive used for thickening, usually derived from corn, sorghum, wheat, or rice

Intake

- US average is 21% of total calories (1979), previously 38% of total calories (1909–1913)
- Recommended intake is at least 48% of total calories or 125 g/ 1000 kcal.

Deficiency Consequences

- Very-low-carbohydrate diets (below 50 g/d) cause increased ketone formation, which may lead to dehydration and mineral depletion. Breakdown of tissue proteins may also occur.

Health Benefits

- Associated with low-fat, low cholesterol, low-calorie, high-fiber diets that have significant health benefits such as
  1. lowered serum triglycerides and serum cholesterol
  2. improved glucose tolerance in diabetes
  3. lowered blood pressure in hypertension
  4. lowered serum estrogens

Carbohydrates and Athletic Training

See Chapter 25, "Sports Nutrition."

GLYCEMIC INDEX

See Appendix C.

CLINICAL MEASUREMENT

See also Chapter 6, "Diabetes Mellitus," and Chapter 14, "Hypoglycemia and Related Disorders."

Urinary Glucose

- Normally absent, its presence indicates severe diabetes due to high renal threshold for glucose.

Fasting Plasma Glucose

- Detects established diabetes when above 140 mg/dL on two occasions.

- Levels over 115 mg/dL indicate possible impaired glucose tolerance.
- May detect fasting hypoglycemia below 60 mg/dL.

Postprandial Plasma Glucose

- Measured after a meal.
- Above 140 mg/dL after 2 hours is abnormal; over 200 mg/dL confirms diabetes.
- No consistent relationship to symptoms in so-called reactive hypoglycemia. See Chapter 14, "Hypoglycemia and Related Disorders."

Oral Glucose Tolerance Test

- fasting plasma glucose followed by 75 g of glucose load and glucose determinations every half-hour
- currently used less often or in abbreviated form (fasting and 2-hour glucose only)

Glucose-Insulin Tolerance Test

- Establishes etiology of glucose intolerance.
- Insulin levels are measured at the same time as glucose during a full glucose tolerance test.

Glycosylated Hemoglobin A_{1c} (Glycohemoglobin)

- Used in diabetes screening and monitoring.
- Hemoglobin in red blood cells irreversibly binds large amounts of glucose during periods of elevated blood sugar.

- Because of the long life span of RBCs, glycohemoglobin levels reflect long-term (about 60 days) control of blood sugar levels.
- Normal glycosylation is less than 5%. Over 7.5% glycosylation is suggestive of diabetes.

Serum Fructosamine

- A test similar to glycohemoglobin, it reflects glycosylation of serum proteins.
- Reflects intermediate term (2 to 3 weeks) control of blood sugar levels.

34. Dietary Fiber

TOTAL DIETARY FIBER

- Dietary fiber includes insoluble and soluble components, which have different effects on human physiology.
- Crude fiber is an obsolete term used when food fiber analysis was done with primitive techniques.

Occurrence

- natural foods: average 3 parts insoluble to 1 part soluble
- beans and peas: 2 to 12 g per serving
- bran breakfast cereals: 4 to 13 g per serving
- fruits with edible skin and/or seeds, oranges, dried fruit: 2 to 4 g per serving
- most vegetables: 2 to 4 g per serving
- cooked whole grains: 2 to 3 g per serving
- whole-grain bread products: 1.5 to 2 g per serving
- nuts and seeds: 1.5 to 3 g/oz
- wheat bran: 1.6 g/Tbs; rice bran: 1.1 g/Tbs; oat bran: 0.8 g/Tbs.

Intake

- US intake is estimated to average 12 g/d.
- Recommended intake is 25 to 35 g/d (National Cancer Institute and others) or 12 g/1000 kcal of dietary intake; some authorities suggest more, up to 20 to 30 g/1000 kcal.

INSOLUBLE FIBER

Occurrence

- abundant in most grains and fibrous fruits and vegetables
- over 6 g per serving—100% wheat bran cereal, figs, raspberries
- 3 to 4 g per serving—most other dried fruit, berries with seeds, winter squash
- 2 to 3 g per serving—whole grains and cereals (including oats and oat bran), asparagus, Brussels sprouts, cooked corn, peas
- 1 to 2 g per serving—whole-grain bread, most other fruit and vegetables with edible skin
- less than 1 g/per serving—most other fruits, vegetables, nuts

Clinical Applications

- Increases fecal bulk, decreases intestinal transit time, reduces intraluminal and intra-abdominal pressures, may alter bacterial flora in colon.
- Helps prevent and alleviate **constipation** (25 to 50 g/d with 1 to 2 qt of additional fluids and vigorous exercise to tolerance).
- Indicated for prevention and treatment of **diverticulosis** (40 g/d).
- May help prevent **colon cancer** by improving general health of intestinal mucosal, by diluting potential carcinogens and speeding their elimination; 22 g/d has caused regression of precancerous lesions.
- May help prevent **hemorrhoids, varicose veins, hiatal hernia** and **cardiac arrhythmias** by reducing straining pressures during bowel movements.
- Suggested, but not proven, to aid in weight loss by increasing satiety after meals.
- May help pain control and restore normal mucus production and normal bowel habits in **irritable bowel syndrome.**
- Associated with low incidence of **hypertension.**

Clinical Measurements

- Intestinal transit time: Use stool marker (activated charcoal, beet powder, chlorophyll, natural food dyes) taken with meal to determine time from ingestion to elimination. Normal transit time is estimated to be 18 to 48 hours by some authorities.

Supplement Considerations

- Insoluble fiber is available as wheat bran and psyllium husk (psyllium functions as both insoluble and soluble fiber).
- Additional fluids must be consumed with a high-fiber diet.
- Drink 6 oz of water per tsp of wheat bran.

Side Effects/Contraindications

- constipation if water intake not increased
- gas due to bacterial fermentation of fiber (usually temporary)
- cramping and diarrhea if excessive fiber introduced into sensitive gastrointestinal tract or during exacerbations of inflammatory intestinal disease
- contraindicated in bowel obstruction or stenosis
- decreased mineral absorption suggested with insoluble fiber but unproven (Vegetarians eat large amounts of fiber yet have superior mineral status.)

SOLUBLE FIBER

Soluble fiber is available as β-glucan (oats, barley), pectin (apples, carrots), etc.

Occurrence

- abundant in oat products (50% of total fiber) and legumes (30% to 50%); also found in lesser amounts in some fruits and vegetables (1 g or less per serving)
- oat bran (dry)—6 g per cup; cooked oatmeal—1.4 g per serving
- all-bran cereal—1.6 g per serving; Cheerios—0.5 g per cup
- cooked corn—1.5 to 2.4 g per serving; cooked brown rice—0.2 g per serving
- whole wheat bread—0.3 g per slice
- black-eyed peas—3.6 g per serving
- kidney beans, garbanzos—2.5 g per serving; pinto beans, pork and beans—2 g per serving; split peas—1.7 g per serving; lima beans—1.3 g per serving
- lentils—1 g per serving
- dried fruit—2 to 3 g/serving; most whole fruit—less than 1 g per serving
- cooked corn—2 g per serving; kale, cabbage, Brussels sprouts, peas, carrots, yams, zucchini—1 to 1.5 g per serving
- most other vegetables—less than 1 g per serving

Clinical Application

- Delays gastric emptying, increases fecal bulk (not as much as insoluble fiber), normalizes intestinal transit time, slows glucose absorption, binds with bile acids to prevent their resorption and reduce fat absorption, provides absorbable short-chain fatty acids after fermentation by gut bacteria; may alter bacterial flora in colon.
- Helps reduce serum total **cholesterol** and **LDL cholesterol** levels 3% to 10% per daily serving; higher initial cholesterol levels decline farthest.
- Improves **glucose tolerance,** reduces need for insulin, and lowers serum triglycerides in insulin-dependent and non-insulin–dependent diabetics.

- May reduce incidence of **gallstones.**
- May help alleviate simple **diarrhea** or symptoms of **irritable bowel syndrome.**

Supplement Considerations

- Soluble fiber supplements include oat bran (30 to 100 g/d), pectin (15 g/d), guar gum (15 to 20 g/d), and glucomannan and psyllium (10 g/d). Also present in food additives such as locust bean gum and xanthan gum.
- Must be taken with meals for maximal effects on blood sugar and lipids.
- Additional fluids must be consumed with a high-fiber diet.

Side Effects

- Constipation is a problem if water intake not increased.
- Gas due to bacterial fermentation of fiber may cause gastric upset (usually temporary).

35. Lipids and Lipid Factors

OCCURRENCE OF DIETARY FATS

Animal Fats

- red meat, dairy—high in saturated fat and cholesterol
- poultry—moderate in saturated fat and cholesterol
- fish with fins—low in saturated fat and cholesterol, some have high polyunsaturated fats (see "Omega-3 Fatty Acids" below)
- shellfish—low in saturated fat, moderate in cholesterol

Plant Oils (No Cholesterol)

- oils of safflower, sunflower, soy, corn, cottonseed; liquid margarines—high in polyunsaturated fat
- oils of olive, rapeseed (canola), almond, peanut, sesame; certain high-oleic hybrids of sunflower and safflower oil; hydrogenated oils, margarines and shortening—high in monounsaturated fat
- oils of coconut, palm and palm kernel—high in saturated fat

Note: Frying oils absorb cholesterol from chicken, fish, etc.

High-Fat Foods

- fast-food hamburgers, all fried foods, pizza, cheese dishes
- bacon, sausage, many cold cuts and luncheon meats, ribs, steak, canned fish in oil

Table 35-1 US Adult Intake of Fat versus US Dietary Goals (% of Total Calories)

Fat*	1986	1901–1913	Dietary Goals
Total fat	36%	32%	<30%
Saturated fat	13%	13%	<10%
Monounsaturated fat	14%	17%	10%
Polyunsaturated fat	7%		10%

*By food source: meats—42% of total fat intake; milk products—17%; grain products—15%; added fats and sweets—10%; fruits and vegetables—9%; eggs and legumes—7%.

- ice cream, Half & Half, nondairy creamer, most cheese
- doughnuts, sweet rolls, pies, pastries, granola, rich cookies and crackers, potato chips and corn chips
- nuts, seeds, peanuts, avocado, olives
- many salad dressings, mayonnaise

DIETARY FATS AND HEALTH

Essential Fatty Acid Requirements

- linoleic acid—1% to 2% of calories or 3 to 6 g/d
- omega-3 fatty acids—10-25% of linoleic acid intake

Deficiency High-Risk Groups

- fat malabsorption syndromes (cystic fibrosis, pancreatic or biliary disease)

Table 35-2 Percentages of saturated and unsaturated fats in common fats

Source	% Saturated	% Monounsaturated	% Polyunsaturated
Coconut oil	87	11	2
Palm kernel oil	82	16	2
Dairy fat	63	33	4
Beef fat	50	46	4
Palm oil	49	41	10
Pork fat	39	50	11
Chicken fat	30	57	13
Turkey fat	30	47	23
Crisco shortening	27	44	29
Cottonseed oil	26	22	52
Stick soybean oil margarine	21	52	26
Wheat germ oil	19	18	63
Tub corn oil margarine	18	43	39
Peanut oil	17	51	32
Tub soybean oil margarine	16	50	34
Liquid margarine	16	39	45
Hydrogenated soybean oil	15	47	38
Soybean oil	15	27	58
Sesame oil	14	44	42
Olive oil	13	79	8
Corn oil	13	28	59
Tub safflower oil margarine	11	34	55
Sunflower oil	10	25	65
Safflower oil	9	17	74
Almond oil	8	74	18
Canola oil	6	62	32

Clinical Measurement

- Malabsorption may be assessed with serum beta carotene, 5-hour postprandial serum triglycerides, or fecal fat.

Deficiency Consequences

- saturated and monounsaturated fat—none
- omega-6 polyunsaturated fats (linoleic, arachidonic)—dry, scaly skin; hair loss; impaired wound healing (see "Omega-6 Fatty Acids" below)
- omega-3 polyunsaturated fats (linolenic)—animal studies suggest impairment of brain and retina function (see "Omega-3 Fatty Acids" below)

Risks and Benefits of Increased Dietary Fat

- total fat—cancer of the colon, breast, and prostate; atherosclerosis; gallbladder disease
- saturated fat—raises serum cholesterol, lowers HDL and increases thrombosis, leading to atherosclerosis, cardiovascular, and cerebrovascular disease; may worsen symptoms of multiple sclerosis
- monounsaturated fat—no apparent individual risk; may help raise serum HDL
- polyunsaturated fat—moderate amounts may reduce serum cholesterol, lower blood pressure, and prevent abnormal blood clotting, which can otherwise lead to heart attack, stroke, or vascular disorders
- high amounts of omega-6 polyunsaturated fats—may depress serum HDL and contribute to cancer etiology and gallstone formation

UNNATURAL DIETARY FATS

Hydrogenated Fats

- Hydrogenated fats contain *trans* fatty acids as well as increased amounts of saturated fatty acids.
- Hydrogenated fats represent up to 40% of fat content of frying oils, shortenings, margarines, coffee creamers, baked goods, frostings, candy, and snack chips.
- Average US diet contains 5% to 15% of its fat as *trans* fats.
- US human subjects possess up to 6% of their tissue fat as *trans* fats.
- Accumulated *trans* fatty acids in body tissues may contribute to disease processes:
    1. cannot function as essential fatty acids
    2. increase LDL/HDL ratio
    3. may be atherogenic
    4. may interfere with prostaglandin balance
    5. may accumulate in and destabilize cell membranes

Oxidized Fats

- Oxidized fats include oxidized fatty acids and oxidized cholesterol; caused by excessive exposure to heat and air.
- Oxidized fats are produced by frying with unsaturated oils, blackening of meats in cooking, hickory smoking of meats, production of dried egg products. They are *not* produced by microwave cooking.
- Commercial US frying fats have been shown to contain up to 8% of their fat content as oxidized fats.
- Oxidized fats may contribute to disease processes:
    1. may produce carcinogens or other toxic products

2. may be specifically toxic to arterial walls, contributing to atherosclerosis
3. may indirectly contribute to oxygen radical production in the body after ingestion

Artificial Fats

- Olestra is a sucrose polyester that is indigestible. Intake of 14 g/d has reduced absorption of cholesterol.
- Simplesse is a specially processed mixture of egg and milk proteins and water. It contains 1 to 2 calories per gram.

CHOLESTEROL

Sources

- liver—372 mg per serving; eggs—215 mg each
- shrimp—150 mg per serving; sardines—129 mg per serving; crab, lobster—100 mg per serving; clams, oysters—50 mg per serving
  Note: Cholesterol in fish and shellfish may not have the same effects as cholesterol in other foods.
- red meats, dark turkey meat—80 mg per serving; light chicken/turkey meat—65 mg per serving; finfish—60 mg per serving
- ice cream—27 to 49 mg per scoop; regular cheese—28 mg/oz; regular milk—32 mg per serving; low-fat milk—14 mg per serving
- butter—12 mg/tsp; mayonnaise—10 mg/Tbs

US Intake

- average = 600 to 800 mg/d, affected most by egg intake

Recommended Intake

- less than 300 mg/day

Associated Health Risks

- Risks may be similar to saturated fat health risks.
- Some individuals appear to tolerate dietary cholesterol well.

High-Risk Groups

- see Chapter 12, "Hypercholesterolemia and Related Lipid Disorders"
- strong cardiovascular risk factors along with moderate increases in serum total cholesterol (>200 mg/dL) and LDL cholesterol (>130 mg/dL)
- serum total cholesterol levels above 240 mg/dL or LDL cholesterol levels above 160 mg/dL regardless of other risk factors
- within lower ranges of intake (0 to 500 mg/d), 100 mg of dietary cholesterol may raise serum cholesterol by 5 to 10 mg/dL in sensitive individuals (This is *not* as powerful an effect on serum cholesterol as is dietary saturated fat.)

Therapeutic Considerations

- Studies demonstrate that lowering blood cholesterol by reducing diet achieves 10% to 15% average reduction in serum levels, although there is wide variation between individuals. Effects are more dramatic from 500 mg/d cholesterol toward zero.
- Effect of reducing dietary cholesterol is minimal when total and saturated fats are already low.

DIETARY FAT AND CHOLESTEROL SCORE

The dietary fat and cholesterol score system was devised in the late 1970s for use in a large, nationwide study of diet and heart disease (MRFIT). The formula used was:

$$\text{Score} = (0.475 \times \text{grams of saturated fat}) - (0.5 \times \text{grams of polyunsaturated fat}) + (0.02 \times \text{milligrams of dietary cholesterol})$$

It seems that these researchers considered 1 g of saturated fat as hazardous as about 24 mg of cholesterol. They also appear to believe that 1 g of polyunsaturated fat more than cancels out the hazardous effect of 1 g of saturated fat.

Research since that time has revealed hazards of excess polyunsaturated fat (see previous section) and questions whether the hazard of dietary cholesterol is the same in different people. Nevertheless, this scoring system may be useful in quickly analyzing a patient's diet for certain excesses.

9 Points

- jumbo fast-food hamburger (Big Mac, Whopper, etc.)

6 Points

- double or quarter-pounder fast-food hamburger

5 Points

- 1 cup meat stew, meat pie, chili, hash, etc.
- 1 cup macaroni and cheese; 1/2 cup lasagna, parmigiana
- two slices cheese pizza (other toppings extra, see below)

- 4 cups popcorn prepared in tropical oil
- one egg or egg yolk

4 Points

- fast-food roast beef or ham sandwich
- one serving of Danish, cheesecake, cream pastry, or pie
- one serving of pound cake, sponge cake, fruitcake, jelly roll
- 1/2 cup custard, rice pudding, bread pudding

Note: Each meat serving below is for a 2-oz (small) portion.

3 Points

- regular fast-food hamburger, meatballs, meatloaf, thick meat sauce, liver, regular cold cuts, frankfurters, sausage, ham, Canadian bacon, most pork and lamb cuts except as noted below
- fatty beef cuts—hamburger, ribs, club/porterhouse/rib/T-bone steak, prime rib
- two pieces fast-food fried chicken
- most cheeses—one slice jack, Swiss, American, Muenster, etc.; 2 Tbs cheese spreads or dips
- 1/2 cup high-fat ice cream (Haagen-Daz, etc.)
- 1 cup whole-milk dairy product (milk, yogurt, etc.)

2 Points

- leaner beef trimmed of fat—round/sirloin/tenderloin cuts, rump or chuck roast, stew meat, extra-lean ground round
- leaner lamb trimmed of fat—chops, leg of lamb
- leaner pork trimmed of fat—boiled/smoked/center-cut ham, pork loin

- veal, poultry with skin (not fried), fried seafood, canned fish in oil
- 1/2 cup regular cottage cheese, regular ice cream, pudding, tapioca
- 1 Tbs cream cheese, sour cream, rich cheese salad dressing
- One slice/2 Tbs lower-fat cheese—mozzarella, ricotta, etc.
- 1 cup low-fat milk dairy product, 2 Tbs whipped cream
- 1 tsp or one pat butter, stick margarine, shortening, tropical vegetable oil
- one serving of rich coffee cake, sweet roll, donut, pancakes (2), waffle, French toast, frosted cake, candy bar, granola bar, double-crust fruit pie, granola with oil (1/2 cup)
- 1/2 cup batter-fried vegetables (tempura), onion rings, fried rice
- 20 thin French fries, 20 small/10 large potato/corn/tortilla chips with tropical oil
- 1 cup thick meat soup, creamy chowders

1 Point

- one slice of bacon
- one serving of poultry without skin, nonfried fish, canned fish in water
- 1/2 cup low-fat cottage cheese, one slice diet cheese
- 2 Tbs Parmesan cheese, cream or cheese sauce, nondairy coffee creamer
- 1 cup cream soups, poultry soups, fish soups, chow mein/chop suey with meat
- 1 Tbs Half & Half, 1/2 cup ice milk
- 1 tsp cooking fat from meat, bacon, lard
- 2 tsp cooking fat from poultry, solid shortening, soft margarine
- 4 Tbs meat gravy, 8 Tbs poultry gravy
- 1/4 cup Brazil nuts, cashews, peanuts, pistachios, mixed nuts
- 4 Tbs peanut butter, 2 Tbs macadamia nuts, 1 Tbs coconut, 1/2 avocado
- 20 small/10 large potato/corn/tortilla chips with nontropical oil

- one serving of muffins, biscuits, rich crackers (12 Ritz, cheese, etc.), unfrosted cake, cookies, brownies, creamy candies, creamy candy sauces

Individuals with high risk to atherosclerotic disease should have diets that score 3 points or below per day in order to minimize the hazards of saturated fat and cholesterol in the diet. Those with moderate risk should score 6 points or below, and those with low risk should maintain a prudent diet that scores 12 points or below.

PLANT STEROLS

Phytosterols

- may compete with cholesterol for intestinal absorption
- β-sitosterol, 300 mg/d with meals, has some effect

OMEGA-3 FATTY ACIDS

- Eicosapentaenoic acid (EPA) and docasahexaenoic acid (DHA) are the most important of the omega-3 fatty acids.

Occurrence

- found primarily in finfish and fish oils
- high-fat fish from cold-water environments, eg, salmon, mackerel, sardines, herring, albacore tuna, brook trout, lake trout, sablefish/black cod, grayfish shark, sturgeon
- fatty fish contain 3 to 12 g of omega-3 oils per pound depending on species, size, age, and environment

US Intake

- estimated at less than 0.25 g/d
- consumption in Japan estimated at 1 to 3 g/d
- consumption by Greenland Eskimos estimated at 6 to 12 g/d

Therapeutic Research

- Substitution of fish oils for more typical dietary plant and animal fats has been found to reduce serum **triglycerides** 45% to 64%, possibly reduce serum **cholesterol** (conflicting studies), and reduce **platelet adhesion.**
- Cholesterol lowering effect not seen when triglycerides are normal.
- MaxEPA, 5 to 10 g/d (20 to 40 mL), or salmon oil, 10 to 15 g/d, provide therapeutic doses but do not have as dramatic an effect on serum lipids as indicated above unless other dietary fats are restricted.
- Salmon and tuna oils, highest in DHA, more consistently produce favorable serum cholesterol changes, whereas pollock oil, highest in EPA, has been shown to *raise* LDL.
- Total omega-3 fatty acids, 5 g/d (3.3 g/d EPA), has reduced elevated **blood pressure;** 1.8 g/d EPA was not effective.
- MaxEPA, 10 to 15 g/d (1.8 to 2.7 g of EPA), plus a low-saturated-fat diet has been shown to relieve some symptoms of **rheumatoid arthritis** and signs of **systemic lupus erythematosus (SLE).**
- MaxEPA, 15 g/d for 6 weeks, reduced **migraine headaches.**
- MaxEPA, 10 g (1.8 g of EPA), reduced severity of **atopic dermatitis** and **psoriasis.**
- Associated with improved weight gain and longer remissions in **ulcerative colitis** and **Crohn's disease.**
- Possible role in managing autoimmune diseases of the kidneys.

Supplement Considerations

- Fish oil products are mixtures of omega-3 and non–omega-3 fatty acids. Labeled content of EPA and DHA should be used to compare potencies.
- MaxEPA (1-g perles) is a proprietary product used in many research studies; 1000 mg contain 300 mg of omega-3 fatty acids (180 mg of EPA and 120 mg of DHA).
- Cod liver oil contains 4 g of omega-3 oils in 25 mL. However, this much oil also contains 7500 IU of vitamin D (toxic) and 25,000 IU of vitamin A.
- α-linolenic acid from flaxseed oil may not be significantly converted in humans to EPA or DHA.

Side Effects/Toxicity/Contraindications

- Omega-3 fatty acids are contraindicated in diabetics due to increases in glucose intolerance.
- Increased bleeding time has been demonstrated in humans; stroke risk is apparently not affected.
- MaxEPA perles contain 6 mg of cholesterol per gram.
- Regular intake of large amounts increases need for vitamin E and, possibly, selenium.

OMEGA-6 FATTY ACIDS

- Linoleic acid is the parent compound of this family. Certain plants contain γ-linolenic acid (GLA), which may have special therapeutic properties.
- Evening primrose oil—9% GLA; black currant seed oil—16.5% GLA; borage seed oil—24% GLA.
- Source: available only in supplement form.

Therapeutic Claims

- Omega-6 fatty acids are recommended for relief of symptoms of prostaglandin-mediated disorders, including inflammatory diseases of many types, allergies, dysmenorrhea, premenstrual syndrome, etc.
- There is very little experimental support for most claims made; there is some evidence of no effect in skin disorders.
- GLA, 540 mg/d, improved symptoms and reduced need for medications in **rheumatoid arthritis.**

Supplement Considerations

- The therapeutic dose range for GLA is 270 to 750 mg/d.
- Up to 2 months of use is required for maximal effects.
- Restriction of dietary saturated and *trans* fatty acids may enhance effectiveness.
- Efamol brand (packaged by many wholesalers), used in most research studies, is considered to be of most reliable potency.

Side Effects/Toxicity/Contraindications

- Allergic reactions are possible but not documented.
- There are some reports of adverse effects in temporal lobe epilepsy and manic-depressive disorder.
- Regular intake of large amounts increases need for vitamin E and, possibly, selenium.

CHOLINE

- occurs in diet as free choline and lecithin or phosphatidylcholine, which is 10% pure choline; synthesized in humans

US Intake

- Average intake is 600 to 1000 mg/d choline from dietary choline *and* lecithin.
- One researcher claims actual intake averages 300 mg/d.

Possible Increased-Need Groups

- Deficiency may contribute to liver cirrhosis in alcoholics.

Therapeutic Research

- Lecithin has long been considered effective in reducing serum cholesterol, but recent literature reviews have concluded that the polyunsaturated fats in lecithin, not the choline, are responsible for the effect.
- Phosphatidylcholine has a slight hypotensive effect in humans.
- One study using a supplement containing 1000 mg of phosphatidylcholine and 4000 mg of high-grade lecithin lowered mortality rates for advanced **atherosclerosis.**
- Phosphatidylcholine, 10 to 30 g/d or choline chloride, 5 to 10 g/d may help improve **short-term memory,** especially in senile individuals.
- Effectiveness of above protocol in reducing symptoms of **Alzheimer's disease** depends on adequacy of acetylcholine synthesis enzyme, which deteriorates as disease progresses.
- Phosphatidylcholine, 10 to 30 g/d, has improved the effectiveness of lithium in manic disorders.
- Phosphatidylcholine may help control other, more rare, neurologic disorders such as **tardive dyskinesia.**
- Treatment of neurologic problems was more effective if cholinergic stimulants were given along with choline.

- Phosphatidylcholine, 1.8 to 3.0 g/d, reduced recovery time in **viral hepatitis.**
- Animal studies demonstrating increased bile solubility with phosphatidylcholine supplementation suggest potential usefulness in gallstone prevention. Preliminary human studies suggest several grams per day would be necessary.

Supplement Considerations

- Commercial lecithin may be only 20% or less phosphatidylcholine.
- Pure phosphatidylcholine used in research is not generally available without a prescription. Supplements labeled phosphatidylcholine are higher-grade lecithin products with over 50% phosphatidylcholine.
- Nonphospholipid choline products (choline bitartrate, choline chloride) contain labeled choline contents but may not have comparable absorption or therapeutic benefits.

Toxicity/Side Effects/Contraindications

- More than 1000 mg of inorganic choline has been associated with nausea, dizziness, depression, and production of a fishy body odor.
- Phosphatidylcholine doses of 20 to 30 g/d are usually well tolerated.

INOSITOL

Sources

- available in diet as *myo*-inositol and phosphatidylinositol
- synthesized in humans

- cantaloupe—355 mg per quarter; orange—307 mg each
- whole-wheat bread—288 mg per slice; 1/2 grapefruit—200 mg
- also in beans, other grains, and nuts

US Intake

- 300 to 1000 mg/d from diet

Possible Increased-Need Groups

- diabetics, patients with multiple sclerosis

Therapeutic Research

- no proven effect on serum cholesterol or heart disease
- 1000 mg/d in addition to the diet in two studies improved nerve function in patients with **diabetic peripheral neuropathy**

Supplement Considerations

- *myo*-Inositol is the only concentrated source of supplemental inositol.

Toxicity/Side Effects/Contraindications

- Malabsorption of large doses may cause diarrhea.

CARNITINE

- structurally similar to choline but not associated with phospholipid molecules in nature; functions as carrier of fatty acids into mitochondria

Sources and US Intake

- Diet provides an average of 100 mg/d from animal foods only.
- Synthesized in humans from lysine using methionine, iron, ascorbate, niacin, and vitamin B6 as cofactors.

Possible Increased-Need Groups

- infants fed soy formulas, possibly strict vegetarians

Deficiency Research

- found in genetic diseases and other conditions
- muscle weakness, cardiomyopathy, hypoglycemia

Therapeutic Considerations

- 2 g/d improved exercise tolerance in **angina pectoris.**
- 4 g/d increased walking distance in **intermittent claudication.**
- Uncontrolled studies have demonstrated reduction of serum triglycerides and raising of HDL cholesterol.

Supplement Considerations

- L-Isomer, not DL mixture, is safest and most effective, but costly.

Toxicity/Side Effects/Contraindications

- DL-Carnitine has caused muscle weakness in some kidney patients on dialysis.
- L-carnitine, 1.6 g/d for over 1 year, has produced no long-term side effects.

36. Protein

SOURCES

- animal flesh foods—15 to 25 g per serving depending on fat content; dairy products—7 to 10 g per serving; eggs—6 g each
- legumes—7 to 8 g per serving; grain products—2 to 3 g per serving; vegetables/fruits—1 to 3 g per serving

RECOMMENDED INTAKE

- Adult RDA = 0.37 g/lb of ideal body weight for height; average man—54 g/d; average woman—45 g/d.
- Athletes may require up to twice RDA levels. See Chapter 25, "Sports Nutrition."
- Pure vegetarian requirements may be approximately 10% higher because of digestibility differences.
- Dietary goals: 8% to 12% of total dietary calorie intake (30 g/1000 kcal).
- Essential amino acids need to make up only about 12% of total dietary protein.
- Upper limit for long-term safety: twice the RDA.

US INTAKE

- 14% to 18% of total daily calorie intake
- adult men—40 to 200 g/d (100 g/d average); adult women—20 to 120 g/d (65 g/d average)

- typical breakdown by food source: 48% meat, fish, poultry; 17% dairy; 16% to 20% grains; 4% eggs
- lacto-ovovegetarians—typically consume 80% of nonvegetarian intake
- pure vegetarians—70% of nonvegetarian intake (1966 data); no evidence of amino acid imbalances in these diets if a variety of sources (grains *and* legumes) are used
- limiting amino acid—methionine (however, intake is still more than twice the minimal requirement in pure vegetarians using a variety of sources)

DEFICIENCY-RISK GROUPS

- uncommon in US except in cases of hypermetabolic disease (systemic cancer, protein-losing enteropathies), severe malabsorption, and trauma (extensive burns)
- athletes on calorie-restricted diets
- possibly those using low-quality proteins exclusively

DEFICIENCY SIGNS AND SYMPTOMS

- edema, muscle wasting, hair loss
- usually occurs as combined protein/calorie malnutrition

CLINICAL MEASUREMENT

- serum albumin for long-term balance
- serum transferrin, prealbumin, or retinol-binding protein for short-term fluctuation
- urinary nitrogen may reflect amino acid breakdown due to excess intake or muscle metabolism

THERAPEUTIC RESEARCH

- Severe **trauma** and **protein-losing pathologies** increase daily requirements to 1.5 to 2.0 g/kg of body weight.
- Low-protein diets reduce deterioration in **chronic renal disease.**

CONSEQUENCES OF EXCESS

- Excess is dangerous in active liver or kidney disease; chronic excess in healthy people is suggested but not proven to be hazardous. Animal studies demonstrate increased risk of renal glomerular sclerosis with aging.
- There is increased calcium loss in urine at higher protein intakes if phosphorus intake is not elevated as well. The typical US diet is not a problem.
- Above 20% of total calories, protein may have tumor-enhancing effects.
- Undigested protein may nourish putrefactive bacteria in colon, allowing exotoxins to be produced in greater amounts. This may be detected with the urinary indican test.
- High-protein diets interfere with the effectiveness of L-dopa in Parkinson's disease.

SUPPLEMENT CONSIDERATIONS

- Supplements are available as whole protein products, partially digested protein products, hydrolyzed amino acids, and free amino acids.
- Predigested or amino acid supplements are often used in allergy elimination diets and malabsorption syndromes.
- Athletes and body-builders frequently consume many times the normal daily requirement, often employing supplemental protein powders.

37. Amino Acids

LYSINE

Estimated Average Requirements

- 5.5 mg/lb of body weight

US Intake

- 3.7 to 8.3 g/d from diet

Therapeutic Research

- **Herpes simplex:** 1 to 3 g/d reduced the frequency of attacks in some, not all, well-controlled studies.

Supplement Considerations

- Supplement is usually given with low-arginine diet (restricted intake of peanuts, nuts, seeds, chocolate).

Toxicity/Side Effects/Contraindications

- Large doses may stimulate cholesterol synthesis.

TRYPTOPHAN

Estimated Average Requirements

- 1.4 mg/lb of body weight

US Intake

- 1.0 to 1.5 g/d from diet

Therapeutic Claims

- **Insomnia:** Tryptophan appears to be effective in mild cases of sleep latency and jet lag. Advise 1 to 3 g taken with a high-carbohydrate/low-protein snack 45 to 60 minutes before bedtime.
- **Pain sensitivity:** 3 g/d with a high-carbohydrate diet may be effective in moderate but not severe pain.
- **Emotional/personality disorders:** There is limited evidence requiring further study in treatment of depression, mania, and aggressive behavior.
- **Depression:** Patients with carbohydrate cravings and high levels of urinary norepinephrine metabolites may benefit from 1 to 3 g/d with a high-carbohydrate/low-protein diet.

Supplement Considerations

- Ingestion along with carbohydrate source enhances brain uptake.
- Except in insomnia, doses should be divided to maintain serum levels.

Toxicity/Side Effects/Contraindications

- A dose of 4 to 5 g/d may cause liver damage.
- Tryptophan is contraindicated in patients taking fluoxetine hydrocholoride (Prozac) and related antidepressants.
- There are reports of fatigue and reduced vigor with tryptophan therapy.
- Tryptophan was recently implicated in an outbreak of eosinophilia-myalgia syndrome, in which 99% of the victims were users of tryptophan supplements. Batch contamination appears to have been the causative factor.

PHENYLALANINE/TYROSINE

Estimated Average Requirements

- 7.3 mg/lb of body weight

US Intake

- 7 to 10 g/d from diet
- diet soft drinks with aspartame sweetener—less than 100 mg of phenylalanine per 12 oz

Therapeutic Research

- **Depression:** Phenylalanine, 2 to 3 g/d, or tyrosine, 100 mg/kg of body weight, may benefit those who also experience lethargy but not carbohydrate craving and excrete low levels of urinary norepinephrine metabolites.

- Tyrosine, 3200 to 4000 mg/d for 6 months, improved symptoms of **narcolepsy.**
- Preliminary reports indicate successful treatment of **cocaine abuse** with tyrosine in conjunction with tryptophan.
- Preliminary reports indicate effectiveness in **stress reduction.**
- May raise *or* lower blood pressure under different circumstances.
- There are unconfirmed claims regarding **appetite suppression.** Over-the-counter appetite suppressants (Dexatrim, Dietac, etc.) contain a more effective derivative of phenylalanine.
- The D isomer of phenylalanine appears to inhibit degradation of natural endorphins, producing relief from **chronic pain** at doses of 600 to 800 mg/d.

Supplement Considerations

- Vitamin B6 supplementation may enhance conversion to neurotransmitters.
- DL-Phenylalanine is a more widely available source of the D isomer, although twice the dosage or more is necessary.

Toxicity/Side Effects/Contraindications

- Contraindicated in patients taking antidepressant drugs containing monoamine oxidase (MAO) inhibitors.
- Contraindicated in patients with malignant melanoma.
- Phenylalanine contraindicated in patients with phenylketonuria (PKU).
- May trigger migraines in those who are prone to them.
- May aggravate rheumatoid arthritis and related disorders.
- Aspartame sweetener may cause headaches, dermatitis, and neurologic symptoms in sensitive individuals. There is some concern over possible fetal toxicity.

SULFUR-CONTAINING AMINO ACIDS

- methionine, cysteine, glutathione (cysteine-containing tripeptide)
- see also "Taurine" below

Estimated Average Requirements

- 4.5 mg/lb of body weight

US Intake

- 2.7 to 4.3 g/d from diet

Therapeutic Research

- Methionine has theoretical, but unproven, benefits as a lipotropic similar to choline. Also unproven are claims for a heavy metal detoxification effect.
- Cysteine and glutathione are established antioxidants and may assist in the elimination of **environmental toxins.** No studies exist on the effects of supplemental doses in humans, however.

Supplement Considerations

- Vitamin B6 is required for many of the interconversions of these amino acids.
- Glutathione has been shown to be absorbed intact at doses of 1 g/d.

Toxicity/Side Effects/Contraindications

- Cysteine is contraindicated in patients with history of cystine kidney stones. High vitamin C may minimize this risk.
- Diabetics taking cysteine should be monitored for decreased glucose tolerance.

TAURINE

- nonessential amino acid synthesized from methionine or cysteine

Occurrence

- found in flesh foods and mother's milk

US Intake

- 40 to 400 mg/d

Possible Increased-Need Group

- infants fed cow's milk formula

Therapeutic Claims

- Taurine is active in bile acid synthesis, neurotransmission, and heart muscle function. It may be useful in related diseases. See Chapter 5, "Cardiovascular Disorders."
- 6 g/d has reduced blood pressure in **hypertension.**

- 3 to 6 g/d has been shown to increase bile acid pool size, which may prevent or reduce **gallstones.**
- Taurine is reported to have mild anticonvulsant effect in **epilepsy** at 500 to 3000 mg/d.

Toxicity/Side Effects/Contraindications

- High doses may have a depressant effect.

ARGININE/ORNITHINE

Estimated Average Requirements

- only semiessential

US Intake

- approximate estimate—5 g/d from diet

Therapeutic Claims

- Suggested to reduce body fat and build muscle based on stimulation of pituitary growth hormone, which has been shown only in animals. Only minor effects have been demonstrated in humans taking large doses.
- Large amounts reduce muscle wasting and accelerate wound healing after **trauma** or **surgery.**
- 30 g/d for 1 week in humans dramatically enhanced **lymphocyte activity.**
- Has inhibited many types of **tumor growth** in animals.

- 4 g/d produced increased sperm count and motility in 80% of men with infertility in one, but not other, studies.

Toxicity/Side Effects/Contraindications

- Contraindicated in growing children.
- Large doses have caused nausea and diarrhea in some persons.
- Large doses with a low lysine intake may promote growth of herpes virus.

BRANCHED-CHAIN AMINO ACIDS

Estimated Average Requirements

- leucine—7.3 mg/lb of body weight
- isoleucine—5.5 mg/lb of body weight
- valine—7.3 mg/lb of body weight

Therapeutic Claims

- Used in clinical medicine to help maintain nitrogen balance in patients with **trauma, liver disease,** or **kidney disease.**
- Used by body builders and other athletes based on physiologic role as muscle energy substrate and inhibitors of protein catabolism. See Chapter 25, "Sports Nutrition."
- **Amyotrophic lateral sclerosis:** Daily doses of 12 g of leucine, 8 g of isoleucine, and 6.4 g of valine preserved muscle mass and walking ability for 1 year.

Toxicity/Side Effects/Contraindications

- branched-chain amino acids compete with tryptophan and tyrosine for uptake into the brain

Bibliography for Part III: Macronutrients

Anderson JW. *Plant Fiber in Foods*. Louisville, Ky: HCF Diabetes Research Foundation; 1986.

Austin S. *Clinical Nutrition* (seminar with bibliography). Portland, Ore: Western States Chiropractic College; 1991.

Austin S. *Clinical Nutrition Update* (periodical). Portland, Ore: Bergner Communications.

Bland JS. *Metabolic Update* (audio periodical with biblographies). Gig Harbor, Wash: HealthComm Inc; 1982–1985.

Brown ML, ed. *Present Knowledge in Nutrition*. 6th ed. Washington, DC: International Life Sciences Institute-Nutrition Foundation; 1990.

Buist R, ed. *International Clinical Nutrition Review* (periodical). Sydney, Australia: Integrated Therapies Pty Ltd.

Committee on Diet and Health, Food and Nutrition Board, National Research Council, National Academy of Sciences. *Diet and Health: Implications for Reducing Chronic Disease Risk*. Washington, DC: National Academy Press; 1989.

Ensminger AH, Ensminger ME, Konlande JE, Robson JRK. *Foods and Nutrition Encyclopedia*. Clovis, Calif: Pegus Press; 1983.

Gaby AR, Wright JV. *Nutrition Therapy in Medical Practice* (seminar with bibliography). Los Angeles: Wright/Gaby Nutritional Seminars; 1985.

Kinsella JE. *Seafoods and Fish Oils in Human Health and Disease*. New York: Marcel Dekker; 1987.

Kritchevsky D. Dietary fiber. *Annu Rev Nutr*. 1988;8:301-328.

Langseth L, ed. *Nutrition Research Newsletter* (periodical). Palisades, NY: Lyda Associates Inc.

Mckee G, ed. *Nutrition and the MD* (periodical). Los Angeles: PM Inc.

Monsen ER, ed. *Journal of the American Dietetic Association* (periodical). Chicago: American Dietetic Association.

Senate Select Committee on Nutrition and Human Needs. *Dietary Goals for the United States*. 2nd ed. Washington, DC: US Government Printing Office; 1978.

Shils ME, Young VR, eds. *Modern Nutrition in Health and Disease*. 7th ed. Philadelphia: Lea & Febiger; 1988.

US Department of Health and Human Services. *The Surgeon General's Report on Nutrition and Health: Summary and Conclusions*. Washington, DC: US Government Printing Office; 1988.

Werbach MR. *Nutritional Influences on Illness: A Sourcebook of Clinical Research*. Tarzana, Calif: Third Line Press; 1988.

Werbach MR. *Nutritional Influences on Mental Illness: A Sourcebook of Clinical Research*. Tarzana, Calif: Third Line Press; 1991.

Yetiv JZ. Clinical application of fish oils. *JAMA*. 1988;260:665-670.

Part IV
Micronutrients

38. Vitamins

VITAMIN A—RETINOL

- 1989 adult male RDA: 1000 μg/d retinol equivalents (RE) = 5000 IU/d
- 1 RE = 1 μg of retinol or 6 μg beta carotene

Occurrence

- retinol in animal foods
- beta carotene and other carotenoids in plant foods (approximately one third converted to retinol by humans)

Rich Sources

- 15,000 IU per serving—beef liver
- 7000 IU per serving—carrots, spinach, sweet potato, winter squash
- 1 to 2000 IU per serving—other dark green vegetables, tomatoes, yellow fruit
- 500 IU per serving—butter, margarine
- 250 IU per serving—dairy products

US Dietary Intake

- adult male average—1419 μg/d of RE total, 2.5 mg of beta carotene
- adult female average—1170 μg/d of RE total, 2.0 mg of beta carotene

- common sources—liver, carrots, eggs, tomato products, vegetable soups, milk products, fortified foods, and supplements

Deficiency High-Risk or Increased-Need Groups

- decreased absorption: alcoholics, children with cystic fibrosis
- decreased beta carotene conversion: hypothyroid, diabetics
- impaired mobilization: liver disorders; protein, iron, or zinc deficiency
- increased utilization: smokers, diabetics, traumatized and infected patients

Deficiency Consequences

- Low carotenoid intake is associated with up to eight times increased risk of some cancers, including lung, oral, gastrointestinal, breast, bladder, cervical, and prostate cancer.
- Low carotenoid intake is associated with increased risk of senile cataracts and chronic pulmonary diseases.
- Low carotenoid intake is associated with increased susceptibility to infections in mucous membranes.
- Classic signs of deficiency include night blindness and dryness of eyes and skin as deficiency worsens.

Clinical Measurement

- Serum retinol reflects adequate tissue availability.
- Dark-adaptation testing is used in research settings.

Therapeutic Research

- **Cancer prevention** effects are seen beginning at a beta carotene dose of 15,000 IU/d (9 mg/d). Larger doses (up to 100 mg of beta carotene) may give increasing protection. Other carotenoids (eg, lycopene) may be equally or more effective.
- **Cancer treatment** using hundreds of thousands of international units of retinol or synthetic derivatives may be useful. There is insufficient research using carotenoids.
- Improved **immune function** may be achieved with short-term doses of 300,000 IU/d or more of retinol or up to 60 mg/d of beta carotene.
- A dose of retinol, 150,000 IU/d for 1 month, improved healing of **gastric ulcers**.
- A dose of retinol, 50,000 IU/d for 2 weeks, may control **menorrhagia.**
- Topical retinoic acid derivatives are effective in controlling **acne** and improving **sun-damaged skin.**
- Oral synthetic retinoid derivatives have improved even severe forms of **acne.** Potentially toxic doses of retinol have also been effective.
- Oral synthetic retinoid derivatives given for 3 to 4 months improved **psoriasis.**
- Retinol or beta carotene improved wound healing in deficient animals.

Supplement Considerations

- Fish liver oil contains varying amounts of retinol and vitamin D.
- Water-soluble, emulsified, and micellized forms of retinol improve absorption and tissue saturation. They are usually more expensive, however.

- Beta carotene is a safe, inexpensive source for supplemental use. Many authorities recommend exclusive use of beta carotene in vitamin A supplements (6 mg of beta carotene = 10,000 IU = 1000 RE).
- Megadoses of vitamin E (over 600 IU) inhibit absorption of beta carotene when taken simultaneously.

Toxicity/Side Effects/Contraindications

- Retinol at a dose of 50,000 IU/d and above may produce reversible headaches, blurred vision, nausea, hair loss, dermatitis, and joint pain. Chronic excess may lead to liver damage.
- A dose of 25,000 IU/d may increase sensitivity to anticoagulant drugs.
- Total retinol intake above 20,000 IU/d is contraindicated in pregnancy because of an association with birth defects.
- Retinol is contraindicated in patients with chronic kidney failure who are undergoing dialysis.
- No apparent toxicity or teratogenicity exists for beta carotene. Harmless yellow skin pigmentation occurs with high doses.

VITAMIN D—CHOLECALCIFEROL

- adult RDA: 200 IU/d (5 μg/d)
- *Note:* Actual need depends on sunlight exposure.

Occurrence

- synthesized in skin from 7-hydroxycholesterol with ultraviolet radiation
- minimal sun exposure (30 min/d) on face and hands is necessary for adequate synthesis in normal persons

- synthesis may be reduced in winter months, in darker-pigmented individuals, and with increased atmospheric ozone concentrations

Rich Sources

- fortified milk—400 IU/qt
- cod liver oil—400 IU/tsp; high-fat fish—250 to 800 IU per serving; canned fish—250-500 IU per serving
- fortification may use synthetic vitamin D_2 (ergocalciferol)

US Dietary Intake

Controversial—official estimates for adults range from 50 to 100 IU/d. Other estimates reach as high as 1000 IU/d or more due to

- use of supplements
- high intake of fortified milk, breakfast cereals, breads, margarines, various packaged beverages
- high intake of foods from animals raised on feed supplemented with vitamin D

Deficiency High-Risk or Increased-Need Groups

- premature and breast-fed infants not exposed to sunlight; 10 µg (400 IU) per day required during most of growth years
- strict vegetarians, confined persons, women with closely spaced multiple pregnancies, persons with severe fat malabsorption syndromes, use of long-term epileptic or cortisone medication, regular use of topical sunscreens
- elderly persons, who produce one half of usual amount of active vitamin D hormone (calcitriol), less in presence of diabetes, kidney disease, or osteoporosis; 15% have low blood levels, especially women

Deficiency Consequences

- hypocalcemia, hyperthyroidism in adults
- rickets (children) and osteomalacia (adults) (considered very uncommon today, although elderly patients with hip fractures have measurable demineralization)
- higher risks of **colorectal** and **breast cancer** according to recent studies

Clinical Measurement

- Serum vitamin D reflects intake/synthesis but not activation.
- Serum 1,25-dihydroxyvitamin D_3 (calcitriol) reflects active hormone levels.
- Serum calcium should be monitored if intake exceeds 1000 IU/d.

Therapeutic Uses

- Elderly patients with impaired vitamin D activation may require large doses (five times RDA) or prescription vitamin D hormone.
- Vitamin D is not beneficial in treatment of **osteoporosis** unless actual deficiency exists; however, active vitamin D hormone, 1 µg/d, has been shown to be effective.
- Recent evidence suggests that active vitamin D hormone (calcitriol) may enhance **immunity** and inhibit **tumors.**
- Calcitriol may be beneficial in treatment of **psoriasis.**

Supplement Considerations

- Because of its abundance in the US diet and availability from sunlight, multiple vitamins need not contain large amounts of vitamin D.

- Fish liver oil contains varying amounts of both vitamin D and retinol.

Toxicity/Side Effects/Contraindications

- Large doses are contraindicated in pregnancy because of teratogenic effects.
- A dose of over 2000 IU/d produces hypercalcemia, which may lead to calcification of soft-tissue and kidney stones.

VITAMIN E—TOCOPHEROL

- 1989 adult male RDA: 10 mg/d α-tocopherol equivalents (α-TE) = 10 IU/d *d*-α-tocopherol
- natural *d*-α-tocopherol now termed RRR-α-tocopherol in scientific publications
- Synthetic *dl*-α-tocopherol now termed all-*rac*-α-tocopherol in scientific publications

Occurrence

- 1 Tbs wheat germ oil—36.3 IU
- 10 to 15 IU per serving—sunflower seeds and oil, almonds, wheat germ
- 5 IU per serving—other polyunsaturated vegetable oils, mayonnaise
- 2 IU per serving—dark green vegetables, margarine
- 1 IU per serving—other fruits and vegetables, animal proteins, whole-grain products

US Dietary Intake

- Intake is estimated to be 10.4 to 13.4 IU/d or 7 to 11 mg of α-TE/d.
- Studies of urban populations have demonstrated deficient average serum tocopherol levels.
- One study showed that 45% of affluent elderly consume less than 75% of RDA.

Deficiency High-Risk or Increased-Need Groups

- inhabitants of urban population centers exposed to ozone; smokers
- high-polyunsaturated-fat diet (0.4 mg α-TE required per g of dietary polyunsaturated fat)
- high oxidized fat intake (See Chapter 35, "Lipids and Lipid Factors.")
- high iron intake, excessive aspirin intake
- intense exercise
- persons with high risk of cancer and other diseases of lung, skin, eye, liver, breast, nervous system, and muscle, which may be caused in part by oxidative damage or free-radical pathology
- premature infants
- newborns fed vitamin E-deficient formula
- children with cystic fibrosis or epilepsy
- severe fat malabsorption syndromes

Deficiency Consequences

- hemolytic anemia and various neurologic disorders in humans; rare in adults

Clinical Measurement

- Serum tocopherol should be compared with total plasma lipids: 6 to 8 mg/g of total lipids is adequate.
- Erythrocyte hemolysis test uses hydrogen peroxide to measure resistance of membrane to oxidation.

Therapeutic Research

- 300 to 1600 IU/d for at least 3 months increased peripheral circulation and walking capacity in **intermittent claudication** and **thrombophlebitis.**
- 100 to 400 IU/d reduced **excessive clotting** tendencies.
- Vitamin E appears to be an important protector of serum lipids, which, if oxidized, become highly **atherogenic.**
- 300 IU/d relieved nocturnal **leg** and **foot cramps.**
- 50 to 100 IU/d with 120 mg/d vitamin C lowered the mutagen content of feces.
- 800 IU/d improved **immune response** in healthy elderly persons.
- Vitamin E is associated with reduced risk of certain **cancers.**
- Vitamin E has an antitumor effect in animals with **breast cancer.**
- 600 to 900 IU/d reduced severity of **fibrocystic disease.**
- 400 IU/d reduced symptoms of **premenstrual syndrome.**
- 100 mg/kg/d reduced severity of **retrolental fibroplasia** in premature infants.
- 400 to 3200 IU/d may slow progression of **Parkinson's disease.**
- Vitamin E is associated with reduced risk for **cataracts.**
- There are unproven claims for prevention of premature aging, miscarriage, impotence and infertility, skin disorders.

Supplement Considerations

- Unknown consequences of pollution and current American diet/life style have led many authorities to recommend preventive megadoses of vitamin E (at least 100 IU/d).
- Supplements are available as pure d-α-tocopherol or tocopheryl ester (natural), mixed tocopherols (natural), or dl-α-tocopheryl ester (synthetic).
- Labeled potency in international units refers to active d-α-tocopherol content *only*.
- Mixed tocopherols may have approximately 20% greater potency than the label indicates because of unmeasured active forms.
- Esterified forms (tocopher*yl*) have longer shelf life but require digestion for activity.
- Alcohol forms (tocopher*ol*) can be used topically or as food preservative.
- Aerosol spray for air-pollution protection is being developed.
- Activity is enhanced by vitamin C and selenium.
- Activity is destroyed in gut if vitamin E is taken with inorganic iron or estrogen.

Toxicity/Side Effects/Contraindications

- Effect of long-term ingestion of l-α-tocopherol from synthetic vitamin E is unknown.
- Acute symptoms are reported occasionally at doses above 100 to 600 IU of any type of vitamin E.
- Temporary gastric upsets and delayed wound healing are reported in some persons taking megadoses.
- Vitamin E is contraindicated with anticoagulant medication or coagulation deficiency; may increase need for vitamin K.

- High doses are contraindicated in rheumatic heart disease because of possible increased valve leakage.
- Gradual increase from small initial doses is recommended for hypertensives (monitor blood pressure).

VITAMIN K—PHYLLOQUINONE, MENAQUINONE

- 1989 adult male RDA: 80 µg (1 µg/kg body weight)

Occurrence

- intestinal bacterial synthesis—up to one half of daily requirement
- dark green vegetables and cabbage family—150 to 800+ µg per serving

US Dietary Intake

- estimated at 300 to 500 µg/d from diet

Deficiency High-Risk or Increased-Need Groups

- unsupplemented newborns, excessive anticoagulant medication or megadose vitamin E
- hospitalized elderly persons
- antibiotic therapy, malabsorption syndromes (may cause deficiency if severe and long-term)
- postmenopausal women, who have 50% lower serum levels than premenopausal women

Deficiency Consequences

- increased bleeding time, hemorrhagic disease
- possibly increased bone loss in elderly persons

Therapeutic Uses

- to reverse deficiency or counteract **anticoagulant overdose** (rat poison ingestion)
- possible role in **osteoporosis** prevention

Supplement Considerations

- Vitamin K is not included in most vitamin supplements.
- Alfalfa tablets contain significant amounts.

Toxicity/Side Effects/Contraindications

- A dose of over 500 mg/d has caused allergic-like symptoms.

VITAMIN B1—THIAMINE

- 1989 RDA = 0.5 mg per 1000 kcal consumed at a minimum of 1 mg/d
- 1989 adult male RDA = 1.5 mg/d

Occurrence

- 1.25 mg/Tbs—brewer's yeast

- 0.6 mg per serving—pork
- 0.2 mg per serving—other meats, peas
- 0.1 mg per serving—milk, other legumes, grains (whole and enriched)

US Dietary Intake

- adult male—1.75 mg/d average, range of 0.6 to 3.0 mg/d
- adult female—1.05 mg/d average, range of 0.5 to 1.8 mg/d
- intake decreases with age

Deficiency High-Risk or Increased-Need Groups

- alcohol abusers, persons with malabsorption syndromes and chronic liver disease, elderly persons
- patients taking certain diuretics (furosemide) or heart drugs (digoxin)
- very physically active adults with high carbohydrate intake
- high intake of raw seafood, tea, coffee, nitrite or bisulfite preservatives, chlorinated tap water
- high intake of unenriched refined carbohydrates
- certain rare genetic disorders causing lactic acidosis, ketoacidosis, etc.

Deficiency Consequences

- anorexia, depression, muscle weakness, peripheral paresthesias, mental confusion, impaired glucose tolerance, edema
- eventually cardiac failure and encephalopathy (wet and dry beriberi)

Clinical Measurement

- Urinary thiamine reflects recent intake.
- Erythrocyte transketolase activity measures tissue saturation and enzyme cofactor requirements.

Therapeutic Research

- 100 mg/d is used to treat deficiency in **chronic alcoholics.**
- Rare thiamine-responsive **anemia** requires 100 mg/d.
- Intravenous thiamine pyrophosphate may improve outcome of **myocardial infarction.**
- There are reduced effects of **lead toxicity** in animals.
- There have been some anecdotal reports of successful therapy in various **neuroses** and **anxiety disorders.**
- There are anecdotal claims of effectiveness as an **insect repellent.**
- There are anecdotal claims of reductions in cravings for sweets.

Supplement Considerations

- The theory that all vitamin B complex vitamins must be consumed simultaneously or in ratio to one another has never been proven. However, it may be prudent to take smaller amounts of vitamin B complex and other water-soluble nutrients whenever a large dose of one B vitamin is used, to compensate for increased diuresis.

Toxicity/Side Effects/Contraindications

- None reported at 500 mg/d for 1 month.

VITAMIN B2—RIBOFLAVIN

- 1989 RDA = 0.6 mg/1000 kcal consumed at a minimum of 1.2 mg/d
- 1989 adolescent male RDA = 1.8 mg/d

Occurrence

- 3.5 mg per serving—beef liver
- 0.4 mg per serving—milk, yogurt, brewer's yeast
- 0.2 mg per serving—meats, cheese, eggs, dark green vegetables
- 0.1 mg per serving—oranges, pineapples, grains, legumes

US Dietary Intake

- adult male—2.08 mg/d average, range of 0.8 to 4.0 mg/d
- adult female—1.34 mg/d average, range of 0.4 to 3.0 mg day
- deficiency high-risk or increased-need groups
- elderly persons, urban poor
- malabsorption syndromes, alcoholics
- thyroid disorders, sickle-cell and other anemias
- oral contraceptive use, certain psychiatric and antidepressant medications
- high intake of psyllium, extensive use of products containing boric acid or borate
- very physically active adults (may double RDA)

Deficiency Consequences

- lip, mouth, eye, and genital irritation
- later seborrheic dermatitis and corneal vascularization

- limited evidence of a role for marginal riboflavin deficiency in early senile cataract formation
- associated with esophageal cancer in some populations

Clinical Measurement

- Urinary riboflavin reflects recent intake.
- Erythrocyte glutathione reductase activity measures tissue saturation and enzyme cofactor requirements.

Therapeutic Research

- 5 to 10 mg/d is used to treat deficiency syndromes. Other B vitamin deficiencies usually coexist.
- Vitamin B2 may reverse **precancerous changes** in esophageal cells.

Supplement Considerations

- The theory that all vitamin B complex vitamins must be consumed simultaneously or in ratio to one another has never been proven. However, it may be prudent to take smaller amounts of vitamin B complex and other water-soluble nutrients whenever a large dose of one B vitamin is used, to compensate for increased diuresis.

Toxicity/Side Effects/Contraindications

- None reported; absorption is very inefficient at high doses.

VITAMIN B3—NIACIN, NIACINAMIDE

- 1989 RDA = 6.6 mg of niacin equivalents (NE) per 1000 kcal consumed at a minimum of 13 NE per day
- 1989 adolescent male RDA = 20 NE per day
- 1 NE = 1 mg of niacin or 60 mg of tryptophan

Occurrence

- 7 mg per serving—peanuts, chicken, salmon, tuna
- 3 mg per serving—other meats
- 1.5 mg per serving—grains, potatoes, peas, brewer's yeast

US Dietary Intake

- adult male—25 mg/d average, range of 9 to 49 mg/d
- adult female—15.5 mg/d average, range of 6.5 to 28 mg/d (does not consider contribution of dietary tryptophan, which is partially convertible to niacinamide) (60 mg of tryptophan = 1 mg of niacin)
- total available NE including tryptophan average—41 mg/d male, 27 mg/d female

Deficiency High-Risk or Increased-Need Groups

- isoniazid therapy, carcinoid syndrome, liver cirrhosis, Hartnup's disease

Deficiency Consequences

- skin and gastrointestinal irritation, central nervous system disorders (pellagra)

Clinical Measurement

- Urinary methylnicotinamide reflects recent intake.

Therapeutic Research

Niacin Only

- A dose as low as 1200 mg/d but usually 3000 to 6000 mg/d lowers elevated **serum cholesterol** (15% to 30%) and **serum triglycerides** (up to 52%) while raising HDL (up to 33%). This therapy has been associated with a decrease in heart attack incidence and fatality. It is often the medical treatment of first choice when diet is not effective.
- 100 to 300 mg/d has been suggested for **vasospastic circulation disorders,** but the effect is temporary.
- Some reports suggest that niacin is beneficial in **drug** and **chemical detoxification** programs that also utilize saunas and exercise.
- There are controversial claims for the treatment of schizophrenia and other neuropsychiatric disorders that have not adequately been substantiated.
- There are anecdotal reports of success in aborting migraine headaches when niacin is taken at earliest indication of onset.

Niacinamide

- One orthopedic practitioner has published many papers concerning his success in treating **osteoarthritis** and some cases of rheumatoid arthritis with 900 to 4000 mg/d.

Supplement Considerations

- Supplements are available as both niacin (nicotinic acid) and niacinamide (nicotinamide). Only niacin produces vasodilation and lowers serum cholesterol.
- Niacin should be started at 100-mg doses taken with meals to minimize flushing.
- The theory that all vitamin B complex vitamins must be consumed simultaneously or in ratio to one another has never been proven. However, it may be prudent to take smaller amounts of vitamin B complex and other water-soluble nutrients whenever a large dose of one B vitamin is used, to compensate for increased diuresis.

Toxicity/Side Effects/Contraindications

- Doses of 100 mg or more of niacin (not niacinamide) produce a temporary flushing reaction and, in some cases, headache and lowered blood pressure. Aspirin or antacids are said to minimize this acute effect.
- Within 2 weeks, daily doses no longer produce this reaction.
- Over 1000 mg/d may produce nausea, vomiting, and diarrhea.
- Megadoses of niacin have been associated with increased risk for cardiac arrhythmias and impaired glucose tolerance.
- Large doses may aggravate peptic ulcers, raise serum uric acid levels, or produce laboratory signs of liver injury.
- Sustained (timed)-release niacin may be more hepatotoxic.
- Side effects may be minimized by gradually increasing doses to target levels.

VITAMIN B5—PANTOTHENIC ACID

- 1989 adult RDA = 4 to 7 mg/d

Occurrence

- 0.8 to 1.0 mg per serving—eggs, milk, poultry
- 0.3 to 0.6 mg per serving—beef, pork, ripe cheese, dried fruit
- 0.1 to 0.3 mg per serving—tuna, whole-grain products, hard cheese, legumes, some fruit and vegetables
- synthesized by microorganisms in lower gastrointestinal tract
- pantethine—metabolite of pantothenic acid developed for therapeutic use in Europe

US Dietary Intake

- Estimated range of 5 to 10 mg/d

Deficiency High-Risk or Increased-Need Groups

- Deficiency is extremely rare.
- One study demonstrated that patients with rheumatoid arthritis have lower serum levels of vitamin B5.

Classic Deficiency Symptoms

- tender heels and feet, fatigue, postural hypotension
- signs of other vitamin deficiencies

Clinical Measurement

- Urinary levels reflect recent intake.

Therapeutic Research

- Pantothenic acid, 500 to 2000 mg/d, reduced morning stiffness, disability, and severity of pain in **rheumatoid arthritis.**
- Preliminary animal and human experiments suggest that large doses may increase resistance to stress and boost energy. Human studies found measurable effects at 2000 mg/d but not at 1000 mg/d.
- Improved wound healing has been reported in animals given pantothenic acid.
- There is no evidence of effect of pantothenic acid on graying or loss of hair.
- Pantethine, 600 to 1200 mg/d, reduced **serum cholesterol** (15%) and **triglycerides** (30%). Pantethine may also inhibit **thrombosis** and **cardiac arrhythmias.**
- Pantethine may reduce toxic effects of chronic **alcohol** consumption.

Supplement Considerations

- The theory that all vitamin B complex vitamins must be consumed simultaneously or in ratio to one another has never been proven. However, it may be prudent to take smaller amounts of vitamin B complex and other water-soluble nutrients whenever a large dose of one B vitamin is used, to compensate for increased diuresis.

Toxicity/Side Effects/Contraindications

- diarrhea in some persons at doses of 10 to 20 g/d pantothenic acid

VITAMIN B6—PYRIDOXINE

- 1989 RDA = 0.016 mg per g of dietary protein intake
- 1989 adult male RDA = 2.0 mg/d

Occurrence

- 0.5 mg per serving—banana
- 0.3 mg per serving—meat, poultry, fish
- 0.2 mg per serving—potato, tomato, corn
- 0.1 mg per serving—milk, dark green vegetables
- 0.05 mg per serving—eggs, raisins, grains, cottage cheese
- bioavailability from different foods varies widely

US Dietary Intake

- varies directly with protein intake
- adult male—1.87 mg/d average
- adult female—1.16 mg/d average
- adult women frequently consume less than 70% of the RDA

Deficiency High-Risk or Increased-Need Groups

- pregnancy, early infancy, the elderly, some diabetics
- medications: oral contraceptives, estrogen, some mood elevators and antihypertensives

Micronutrients 275

- alcohol abuse, high-protein diet, high stress
- certain genetic disorders of amino acid metabolism

Mild Deficiency Consequences

- depression due to inadequate serotonin synthesis, especially in oral contraceptive users
- increased oxalic acid production, which may increase risk of kidney stones
- increased homocystine production, which is atherogenic
- decreased tolerance to monosodium glutamate
- possibly impaired ability to regulate blood sugar, especially in pregnant women and oral contraceptive users
- peripheral nerve dysfunction
- immune system depression, especially in elderly

Clinical Measurement

- Urinary levels reflect recent intake.
- Erythrocyte aminotransferase activity measures tissue saturation and enzyme cofactor requirements.
- Urinary xanthurenic acid levels measured after an oral load of tryptophan may show early deficiencies.

Therapeutic Research

- Some types of **peripheral neuropathy** including **carpal tunnel syndrome** have been responsive to 100 to 200 mg of vitamin B6 daily for up to 3 months.
- 500 mg/d for 3 months gave relief from **premenstrual syndrome.** There is limited evidence of benefit from smaller doses.

- 50 to 300 mg/d reduced urinary oxalate excretion in patients susceptible to oxalate **kidney stones.**
- 100 mg/d improved glucose tolerance in pregnant women with **gestational diabetes** in some studies.
- 75 to 600 mg/d reduced symptoms of **nausea** and **vomiting** in pregnant women.
- Vitamin B6 may reduce the need for insulin in **diabetics.**
- One general medical practitioner reported success using vitamin B6 in various forms of **arthritic** and **rheumatic disorders.**
- 400 to 600 mg/d produced clinical improvement in **autism.**
- 5 mg/d is sufficient to counteract effects of **oral contraceptives** on B6-related metabolism.
- There is preliminary evidence that topical pyridoxal cream may cause regression of **malignant melanoma.**
- There is anecdotal evidence that large doses of vitamin B_6 increase conception rates in women with unexplained infertility.
- Vitamin B6 is not recommended for simple edema, since excessive amounts may be necessary.

Supplement Considerations

- Pyridoxal 5-phosphate is hydrolyzed to free vitamin B_6 in the intestine and is therefore not likely to be superior to standard vitamin B6 supplements.
- The theory that all vitamin B complex vitamins must be consumed simultaneously or in ratio to one another has never been proven. However, it may be prudent to take smaller amounts of vitamin B complex and other water-soluble nutrients whenever a large dose of one B vitamin is used, to compensate for increased diuresis.

Toxicity/Side Effects/Contraindications

- Excessive intake (1000 mg/d for 1 year or 2000 mg/d for 2 to 4 months) produced neurologic disturbances such as numbness and motor dysfunction. There are some reports of similar effects from doses as small as 200 mg/d for 6 months or more.
- Vitamin B6 inactivates most forms of L-dopa medication in the intestine; therefore, it is contraindicated in patients with Parkinson's disease being treated with these drugs.

FOLIC ACID

- 1989 RDA = 3 µg/kg of body weight
- 1989 adult male RDA = 200 µg/d

Occurrence

- 300 µg/Tbs of brewer's yeast
- 185 µg per serving—beef liver
- 100 µg per serving—asparagus
- 70 µg per serving—orange, peanuts, beets, spinach
- 50 µg per serving—legumes, broccoli, Brussels sprouts, cantaloupe
- 25 µg per serving—eggs, green leafy vegetables, peas, grapefruit, tomatoes, bananas
- more available forms in some foods than in others
- sensitive to heat, prolonged storage, water; up to 50% typically destroyed before food is consumed
- absorption enhanced by vitamin C

US Dietary Intake

- average intake = 220 µg/d
- in Canada, average intake = 205 µg/d in men and 149 µg/d in women

Deficiency High-Risk or Increased-Need Groups

- decreased intake/absorption: hospitalized patients, others on low fresh-food diets, alcohol abusers, patients with atrophic gastritis and malabsorption syndromes
- increased utilization: pregnancy/lactation, bottle-feeding, proliferative diseases (psoriasis, hemolytic, or sickle-cell anemia), cirrhosis, smoking, increased metabolic rate, vitamin B12 deficiency
- medication interactions: oral contraceptives, anticonvulsants, some antacids, antihypertensives, aspirin

Deficiency Consequences

- megaloblastic anemia, glossitis, gastrointestinal irritation
- depression and other neuropsychiatric disturbances
- spontaneous abortion, cleft palate, birth defects of the neural tube type (occurs in first month of gestation)
- possibly increased risk of chromosome breakage, mutation, and cancer

Clinical Measurement

- Serum folate reflects recent intake.
- Erythrocyte folate reflects tissue stores.
- Macrocytic anemia appears after months of depletion.

- Above tests may be positive in vitamin B12 deficiency also.
- Deoxyuridine suppression test differentiates between folate and vitamin B12 deficiency.

Therapeutic Research

- Supplementation during **pregnancy** decreases incidence of premature birth, small-for-date births, and neural tube defects.
- 10 mg/d for 3 months improved precancerous **cervical dysplasia.**
- 10 mg/d along with vitamin B12, 500 µg/d, reversed possible **precancerous changes** in lung cells of cigarette smokers.
- 5 mg/d improved circulation and visual acuity in elderly **diabetics.**
- Daily doses of either 250 µg or 10 mg have been shown to improve behavior and IQ in some preadolescents with **mental retardation** (fragile-X syndrome).
- Folic acid mouthwashes (5 mg in 5 mL of water) decreased the severity of **periodontal gum disease.**

Supplement Considerations

- Supplemental folate is absorbed twice as well as food folate.
- A dose of up to 1000 µg/d is used in treatment of deficiency.
- Patients should be evaluated for pernicious anemia and vitamin B12 deficiency before being given large doses of folate.

- **Toxicity/Side Effects/Contraindications**

  - Doses of folic acid over 1000 µg can mask the more obvious signs of B12 deficiency.
  - Doses over 350 µg/d may reduce absorption of zinc.

- Large doses are contraindicated for epileptics stabilized on certain anticonvulsants.

VITAMIN B12—COBALAMIN

- 1989 adult RDA = 2 µg/d

Occurrence

- generally available from most animal sources and absent from most plant sources
- 10+ µg per serving—organ meats, clams, oysters
- 2.0 µg per serving—beef, lamb, other seafoods
- 1.0 µg per serving—chicken, eggs, milk, cottage cheese
- 0.5 µg per serving—pork, hard cheese
- reported content may include up to 30% inactive forms of vitamin B12
- present in fermented soybean products and seaweed, but content is variable and includes many inactive forms
- not found in brewer's yeast

US Dietary Intake

- adult male—7.84 µg/d average
- adult female—4.85 µg/d average

Deficiency High-Risk or Increased-Need Groups

- pernicious anemia due to lack of intrinsic factor, achlorhydria, and other malabsorption syndromes (more than 95% of vitamin B12 deficiency syndromes)

- strict vegetarians (especially children and breast-fed infants of vegan mothers), elderly persons, those who have had gastrointestinal surgery
- alcohol abusers, smokers
- no support for claims that high dose vitamin C intake destroys vitamin B12

Deficiency Consequences

- megaloblastic anemia, gastrointestinal irritation
- motor, sensory, and cognitive impairment with or without anemia

Clinical Measurement

- Serum B12 reflects early reduction in tissue stores.
- Macrocytic anemia appears after months or years of depletion.
- Deoxyuridine suppression test differentiates between folate and vitamin B12 deficiency.

Therapeutic Research

- 1000 μg/d prevents deficiency in **pernicious anemia** due to passive 1% to 3% absorption without intrinsic factor function.
- 2000 to 4000 μg sublingually with a meal containing sulfite food (and wine) additives may prevent or diminish headache, upper respiratory, and asthmatic **reactions to sulfite** in susceptible persons.
- 500 μg/d along with megadoses of folic acid reversed possible **precancerous changes** in lung cells of cigarette smokers.
- There is preliminary evidence of benefit to elderly people with **neurologic** or **psychiatric disorders.**
- Anecdotal reports of energy tonic effect have not been adequately researched.

- The theory that vitamin B12 injections can reverse diabetic neuropathy is unproven.

Supplement Considerations

- Resin-bound preparations may have superior absorption.
- There is no conclusive evidence of the superiority of sublingual vitamin B12 preparations.
- Intranasal vitamin B12 may be used in pernicious anemia. Absorption was actually superior to oral doses in one study.

Toxicity/Side Effects/Contraindications

- None reported at doses up to 100 μg/d.

BIOTIN

- 1989 adult estimated safe and adequate daily dietary intake = 30 to 100 μg

Occurrence

- 100 to 200 μg per serving—liver
- 25 to 50 μg/oz—nutritional yeast
- 23 μg per serving—almonds
- 20 μg/oz—soy flour
- 11 μg each—egg yolk
- 4-7 μg per serving—whole-grain breads and cereals
- synthesized by microorganisms in lower gastrointestinal tract

US Dietary Intake

- 28 to 42 µg/d

Deficiency High-Risk or Increased-Need Groups

- infants
- chronic use of antibiotics, very-low-calorie diets
- consumption of large amounts of raw egg white
- achlorhydria

Deficiency Consequences (rare)

- hair loss, scaly dermatitis

Clinical Measurement

- Serum biotin reflects total absorbed vitamin.

Therapeutic Research

- 5 mg/d reversed **seborrheic dermatitis** in deficient infants.

Toxicity/Side Effects/Contraindications

- None reported at intakes up to 10 mg/d.

VITAMIN C

- 1989 adult RDA = 60 mg/d, 100 mg/d for smokers
- tissue saturation occurs at 200 mg/d

Occurrence

- 100 mg per serving—kiwi fruit
- 50 to 65 mg per serving—broccoli, Brussels sprouts, oranges and juice
- 35 to 50 mg per serving—green pepper, grapefruit, strawberries, melons
- 15 to 20 mg per serving—cabbage, asparagus, tomatoes and juice, potatoes, pineapple and juice, spinach, banana, lemon, berries
- sensitive to air and heat

US Dietary Intake

- average adult daily intake from food alone—109 mg (males), 77 mg (females)
- range—10 to 250 mg/d from food alone
- common sources—citrus fruits, tomato products, potatoes, fortified beverages
- primitive humans possibly ingested 300-600 mg/d
- most popular nutritional supplement, used by 35% to 50% of the population

Deficiency High-Risk or Increased-Need Groups

- infants fed only cow's milk, elderly men
- institutionalized populations

- alcoholics, smokers, others exposed to various pollutants
- users of drinking water with chlorine or chloramine additives
- high physical (and, possibly, emotional) stress
- iron-deficient individuals
- chronically ill, surgical, and severely wounded or infected patients; diabetics
- chronic psychiatric patients
- oral contraceptive users, chronic aspirin users

Deficiency Consequences

- Early signs are easy bruising, followed by swollen or bleeding gums and petechial hemorrhages.
- Marginal deficiency is linked with cancer, especially gastric, esophageal, laryngeal, and cervical cancer.
- Marginal deficiency is linked with atherosclerosis, cataract formation, periodontal disease, and one form of male infertility (excessive sperm agglutination).

Clinical Measurement

- Serum ascorbate reflects recent dietary intake.
- Leukocyte ascorbate reflects tissue saturation.
- Lingual test is considered unreliable.

Therapeutic Research

- 25 to 75 mg/d increases nonheme **iron absorption** by two to four times; should accompany all iron-containing meals.
- 500 mg/d or more reduced duration of **common colds** by an average of 37% and also lessened the severity but not usually the frequency of these infections.

- Large doses increased various measures of **immune response** in preliminary studies.
- 120 to 1000 mg/d lowered production of some **carcinogens** in the body.
- Over 90 mg/d helps prevent **cervical cancer**.
- 10,000 mg/d extended survival of **cancer** patients who had not received aggressive medical therapy.
- Two recent short-term controlled trials against human cancer were judged failures but have been criticized.
- 500 to 3000 mg/d lowered serum **cholesterol** in marginally deficient hypercholesterolemic patients.
- 1000 to 2000 mg/d reduced **blood clotting** and **thrombus** formation.
- 500 to 1000 mg dose lessened severity of subsequent exercise- and irritant-induced **asthma** attacks.
- Supplementation reduced free radical production in the lungs of **smokers.**
- 400 mg/d with vitamin E, 400 IU/d, reduced **colon polyp** recurrence.
- 1000 mg/d reversed **infertility** in marginally deficient men with sperm agglutination.
- In combination with a low-vanadium diet, vitamin C improved symptoms in **manic-depressive illness.**
- 500 to 1000 mg/d increased the rate of **wound healing.**

Supplement Considerations

- Dosages above tissue saturation level (200 mg/d) may have effects in the gastrointestinal tract, blood stream, and urinary tract. Many authorities recommend 250 to 1000 mg/d for adults.

Ascorbic Acid versus Mineral (Nonacidic) Ascorbate

- Acid form may lower urinary pH, aggravate gastric lesions.

- Buffered form contributes to mineral intake (about 10% of vitamin C dose).

Normal or Timed/Sustained Release

- Normal release causes rapid peak and decline of serum levels.
- Sustained release is effective for 6 to 8 hour disintegration rate only; longer rates diminish absorption.

With or Without Rose Hips, Acerola, Bioflavonoids

- Added "natural" factors increase cost with no proven benefit. All research studies have used pure vitamin C.

Other Considerations

- Ascorbyl palmitate is a fat-soluble form not found in nature. There is no evidence that this is more beneficial than other fat-soluble antioxidants.
- Sago palm-derived vitamin C may be better tolerated by persons highly allergic to standard corn-derived vitamin C.
- Absorption = 90% of 100-mg dose, 50% of 1000-mg dose.

Toxicity/Side Effects/Contraindications

- Kidney stones are unlikely except in those already prone to stone formation.
- Symptoms of gout are unlikely except in those already suffering from gout.
- Diarrhea may occur when a single dose overloads absorption capacity (usually more than 1000 mg at a time).
- Rebound scurvy after sudden discontinuation of megadoses is documented only in newborns of supplemented mothers.

- Acidic chewable vitamin C tablets have been linked with dental erosion.
- Do not take vitamin C with aspirin (gastrointestinal bleeding) or inorganic selenium (renders selenium non-absorbable).
- Vitamin C interferes with laboratory tests for glucose (false-negative or false-positive) and occult blood (false-negative).

BIOFLAVONOIDS

Occurrence

- Bioflavonoids occur in fresh fruits and vegetables that are high in vitamin C; also found in coffee, tea, cocoa, wine, and beer.
- Commercial sources include rose hips and acerola cherries.
- Bioflavonoids are commercially extracted from citrus pulp and peel and buckwheat leaves.
- Over 500 varieties of bioflavonoids exist.

US Dietary Intake

- estimated at 1000 mg/d average

Deficiency High-Risk or Increased-Need Groups

- possibly those with excessive capillary fragility or permeability, especially if fruit and vegetable intake is low

Deficiency Consequences

- no proven deficiencies in humans; not considered an essential nutrient

Therapeutic Research

- Bioflavonoids are suggested for use in **microcirculatory disorders** such as retinopathy, cerebral hemorrhage risk, menorrhagia, and idiopathic edema or bruising.
- Rutin, 200 to 600 mg/d, decreased **capillary fragility** and **bruising** in humans. Citrus bioflavonoids have similar effects.
- There is preliminary evidence that bioflavonoids, especially quercitin, block synthesis of **inflammatory prostaglandins** and **leukotrienes.**
- There is preliminary evidence that bioflavonoids block reactions that lead to **diabetic cataract.**
- There is preliminary evidence that bioflavonoids stimulate liver enzymes that break down **carcinogens.**
- There is preliminary evidence that quercitin, hesperidin, and catechin have **antiviral** properties.

Supplement Considerations

- Many different members of the family exist: citrin, hesperidin, rutin, quercitin, catechin, etc.
- Therapeutic dose = 500 to 2000 mg/d.
- Bioflavonoids do not appear to enhance effects of vitamin C.

Toxicity/Side Effects/Contraindications

- There is preliminary evidence that quercitin in large amounts is mutagenic.

39. Minerals

BORON

- Estimated safe and adequate daily dietary intake (ESADDI) is unknown.

Occurrence

- high in plant foods, especially fruits, vegetables, nuts, wine, cider, and beer

US Dietary Intake

- average—1.7 to 7.0 mg/d

Deficiency High-Risk or Increased-Need Groups

- possibly individuals at high risk for osteoporosis
- individuals with high risk of magnesium deficiency

Deficiency Consequences

- possibly disturbed metabolism of calcium, phosphorus, and magnesium

Clinical Measurement

- Boron is detectable in hair trace mineral analysis, but the significance is unknown.

Therapeutic Uses

- 3 mg/d in postmenopausal women reduced urinary excretion of calcium and magnesium and increased hormones related to **osteoporosis** prevention.

Supplement Considerations

- Boron is contained in some multivitamin/mineral and bone support products, usually as sodium borate.
- Safe and adequate levels appear to range from 2 to 6 mg/d.

Toxicity/Side Effects/Contraindications

- very low toxicity from oral ingestion up to 20 mg/d

CALCIUM

- 1989 adult RDA = 800 mg/d
- 1989 young adult RDA = 1200 mg/d

Occurrence

- 600 mg per serving—tofu processed with calcium (absorption may not be optimal)

- 400 mg per serving—sardines
- 300 mg per serving—milk, yogurt, buttermilk, milk puddings, canned salmon (with bones)
- 200 mg per serving—hard cheeses (cheddar, American, etc.)
- 150 mg per serving—tofu processed with nigari ($MgSO_4$), blackstrap molasses
- 100 mg per serving—ice cream, ice milk, scallops
- 75 mg per serving—cottage cheese, dark green vegetables

US Dietary Intake

- adult males—850 mg/d average, 200 to 2000 mg/d range
- adult females—500 mg/d average, 135 to 1400 mg/d range
- 30% of population, mostly women, consume less than RDA
- average intake of women over age 40—475 mg/d
- 55% of US calcium intake from dairy products

Deficiency High-Risk or Increased-Need Groups

- small-framed women, especially Caucasian and Oriental, with a long postmenopausal life expectancy
- all elderly individuals, especially those who are intolerant to dairy products, those who are achlorhydric, those who have had surgical removal of the upper gastrointestinal tract, and those on various medications, including cortisone, some diuretics, and aluminum antacids
- those who do not get regular sunshine, vitamin D, or exercise
- those whose diets are high in supplemental protein, which may increase urinary calcium (Typical high-protein, high-phosphorus US diets do not appear to be a problem.)
- those with high intake of phytate from cereal bran or oxalate from spinach and other vegetables, which may reduce calcium absorption

Micronutrients 293

- those who have diabetes, kidney or thyroid disease, or vitamin D metabolism defects, who are at increased risk for osteoporosis
- some additional risk for osteoporosis when diet is high in salt, alcohol, or caffeine
- some additional risk for osteoporosis when diet is low in calories, zinc, copper, fluoride, manganese, silicon, or boron

Clinical Measurement

- Serum total or ionized calcium does not vary with dietary intake or slow bone loss.
- Fasting urinary calcium/creatinine ratio over 0.4 is correlated with osteoporotic bone loss in the absence of gross bone or kidney pathology.
- Hair calcium is less reliable, as it may be high or low in deficient states and is always lower in gray hair.
- Accurate assessment of bone density requires tomographic densitometry or photon absorptiometry techniques.

Deficiency Consequences

- poor development of bones and teeth during growth years
- osteomalacia (severe deficiency) and increased risk of osteoporosis in adults
- possibly contributes to periodontal disease in adults

Therapeutic Uses

- Optimal calcium intake is most important from childhood to young adulthood, when peak bone mass is achieved.
- For normalization of calcium balance and prevention of **osteoporosis** (National Institutes of Health committee recommendations), advise

1. 1000 mg/d for premenopausal women
2. 1500 mg/d for postmenopausal women
3. 1000 mg/d for men over age 40 years

- 1000 mg/d with estrogen replacement in early postmenopausal years was as effective in reducing **bone loss** as higher levels of estrogen alone.
- 1.5 to 2.5 g/d without hormone replacement reduced **bone loss** in women after the fifth postmenopausal year but not during the first 5 postmenopausal years.
- 1000 to 2000 mg/d significantly reduced **blood pressure** 10% to 20% in some hypertensives.
- 2000 mg/d reduced **muscle cramps** in pregnant women.
- There is preliminary evidence of a preventive role against **colon cancer;** 1500 mg/d may provide optimal protection.
- There is no evidence for claims of effectiveness as a natural tranquilizer.

Supplement Considerations

- Tablets should disintegrate in vinegar within one-half hour with occasional stirring.
- Large single doses are much more poorly absorbed than small doses.
- Recent evidence suggests that there may not be much difference in calcium absorption from different foods or supplement sources in amounts up to 500 mg per dose.
- Calcium carbonate (oyster shell, eggshell) is the most concentrated (up to 600 mg per tablet) and inexpensive source. It should be taken with meals to enhance absorption.
- Calcium citrate, lactate, gluconate, chelate, and orotate are considered to be better absorbed (controversial), but the concentration is usually very low (as little as 50 to 100 mg per tablet).

- Recent innovations using calcium citrate-malate and calcium-fortified orange juice appear to demonstrate superior absorption.
- Liquid, powdered, and chewable supplements are better absorbed. Smaller doses are better absorbed.
- There is some evidence that microcrystalline hydroxyapatite has superior absorption and bone-rebuilding effects. See Chapter 22, "Osteoporosis."
- Commercial bone meal contains unneeded phosphorus and possibly lead.
- Dolomite contains poorly absorbed magnesium carbonate and possibly lead.
- A 2:1 ratio of calcium/magnesium content is common and matches RDAs, but the individual's diet composition must be considered.

Toxicity/Side Effects/Contraindications

- Dosages up to 2500 mg/d produce no known side effects in healthy adults.
- High intakes, especially as carbonate or phosphate, may inhibit absorption of iron, zinc, and other minerals.
- The claim that calcium interferes with magnesium absorption only holds for large doses (total of more than 500 mg) taken simultaneously. There is no evidence that calcium intake can cause magnesium deficiency.
- Supplemental calcium is contraindicated in hyperparathyroidism and osteolytic cancer.
- Calcium supplements should be used with caution in persons prone to kidney stone formation or with evidence of hypercalcuria. The citrate form is safest.
- There is no evidence that calcium can contribute to soft tissue calcification in normal persons.

CHROMIUM

- 1989 adult ESADDI = 50 to 200 μg/d

Occurrence

- 20 to 90 μg/Tbs (10 g)—brewer's yeast
- 50 to 60 μg per serving—peanuts
- 20 to 30 μg per serving—poultry, most legumes
- 10 to 15 μg per serving—wheat products, red meats, cheese, most vegetables
- some food tables show erroneously high values due to contamination by stainless steel analytical tools
- stainless steel cookware may provide some utilizable chromium

US Dietary Intake

- estimated intake—27 μg/d, range of 13 to 39 μg/d in one study
- one third of professionally designed optimal diets—less than 50 μg/d

One Canadian study showed that over two thirds of women had less than 50 μg/d in their diets.

Deficiency High-Risk or Increased-Need Groups

- family history or other risk of diabetes
- elderly persons, women with multiple pregnancies
- high sugar diet (increases urinary excretion)
- possibly physical injury or strenuous exercise

Clinical Measurement

- No reliable normal values have been set for urinary or blood levels. Laboratory analysis with stainless steel equipment may contaminate samples.
- Hair analysis requires sensitive equipment but may reveal significant deficiencies.

Deficiency Consequences

- impaired insulin function and glucose tolerance
- elevated serum cholesterol

Therapeutic Research

- Chromium chloride, 200 µg/d, improved **glucose tolerance** in otherwise healthy nondiabetics.
- Patients with mild **diabetes** had 2-hour glucose levels return to normal after chromium supplementation.
- Other studies have shown 50% reductions in fasting serum glucose and 10% reductions in glycosylated hemoglobin.
- Chromium-rich yeast improved impaired **glucose tolerance** in elderly patients.
- Some studies on patients with established diabetes showed no effect, probably because these patients were not chromium-deficient.
- Chromium improved glucose tolerance in patients with **hypoglycemia** as well.
- 200 µg/d in most studies reduced total **serum cholesterol** by 7% to 17% and reduced LDL cholesterol by 11% while slightly raising HDL cholesterol.

- Two studies demonstrated increased **lean body mass** in weight-training athletes and non-athletes taking chromium picolinate, 200 µg/d, compared with placebo.

Supplement Considerations

- Organically bound chromium (as in food) is 15% to 20% better absorbed than inorganic forms (such as chromium chloride).
- Lower doses are required when brewer's yeast or other yeast-bound forms of chromium are used.
- Chromium picolinate and polynicotinate are newly available forms that may have superior bioavailability.
- So-called "GTF chromium" is not a standardized identity and may refer to any organically bound chromium.
- Some suppliers report GTF activity by biologic assay for their product. This is a valid procedure and has shown true GTF complexes (composed of chromium, nicotinic acid, and certain amino acids) to be similar in activity to chromium yeast and three times more potent than other forms of chromium.
- Diabetics taking insulin may experience hypoglycemic reactions if they do not readjust their insulin dosages after taking chromium.

Toxicity/Side Effects/Contraindications

- Of all minerals chromium is one of the least toxic. One therapeutic trial used chromium chloride, 2000 µg/d for 3 months, without toxic effects.
- There are some reports of insulin inhibition at high doses.

COPPER

- 1989 adult ESADDI = 1.5 to 3.0 mg/d
- humans may adapt to less than 1 mg/d without signs of deficiency

Occurrence

- amount in plant sources depends on soil content
- 4 mg per serving—crab
- 3 mg per serving—liver
- 2.3 mg each—oysters
- 0.2 to 0.3 mg per serving—nuts, seeds, most legumes, dried fruit
- 0.05 to 0.1 mg per serving—meats, poultry, seafood, peas, wheat products (may be unavailable due to phytates)

Storing or cooking acidic foods in copper vessels may add significant and, possibly, excessive amounts to daily intake.

Drinking water content is highly variable because it is affected by water pH and plumbing composition.

US Dietary Intake

- average adult intake is 1.2 mg/d (male), and 0.9 mg/d (female)
- 75% of adults consume under 2 mg/d from diet (water supply not taken into consideration, however)

Deficiency High-Risk or Increased-Need Groups

- infants with chronic diarrhea, premature infants
- high intake of zinc, iron, molybdenum

- high intake of bran, fructose
- high intake of vitamin C (1500 mg/d in one study)
- chronic exposure to mercury and cadmium
- elderly persons

Clinical Measurement

- Serum levels reflect recent intake.
- RBC superoxide dismutase is used in research.
- Hair levels do not correlate well with tissue levels in humans, and hair may be contaminated by copper-containing shampoos, hair treatments, and water supplies.

Deficiency Consequences

- iron-deficiency anemia, neutropenia, and impaired connective tissue synthesis in severe deficiencies (rare)
- Menkes' kinky hair syndrome—genetic, fatal by age 3 years
- possible increased inflammatory and oxidative tissue damage (free radical pathology) due to reduced activity of copper-containing antioxidants
- marginal intakes are associated with increased risk of emphysema, cardiovascular degeneration, elevated LDL cholesterol/lowered HDL, and some cancers

Therapeutic Uses

- The use of a copper bracelet for treatment of **rheumatoid arthritis** was validated in one single-blind, placebo-controlled crossover study. Investigators postulated dermal assimilation of copper.

Supplement Considerations

- Copper salicylate (copper aspirinate), once suggested for inflammatory conditions, is no longer available over-the-counter in the United States.
- Copper sulfate, gluconate and chelate have similar bioavailabilities.

Toxicity/Side Effects/Contraindications

- Gastrointestinal upset is reported after single doses of more than 15 mg.
- Wilson's disease (hepatolenticular degeneration) is a genetic disorder of copper accumulation; it usually appears in late adolescence.
- Excessive intake of copper may enhance oxidative tissue damage and also may raise blood pressure.

FLUORIDE

- 1989 adult ESADDI = 1.5 to 4.0 mg/d
- maximal dose = 2.5 mg/d for children, 10 mg/d for adults
- 1.0 mg/L in drinking water

Occurrence

- Seafood: 0.2 to 2.0 mg per serving
- Tea: 0.1 mg per cup

Water supply contributes 0.7 to 1.2 mg/L if adequate fluoride is present.

Sixty percent of US water systems, including most large urban supplies, are fluoridated.

US Dietary Intake

- estimated range—0.2 to 3.4 mg/d depending on soil and water content

Deficiency High-Risk or Increased-Need Groups

- infants on unfortified formula or breast-fed
- children with high exposure of oral cavity to sugars
- those drinking water with less than 0.7 ppm (ask local board of health)
- possibly high osteoporosis risk

Deficiency Consequences

- dental caries
- possibly osteoporosis and early senile hearing loss
- increased incidence of aortic calcification

Therapeutic Uses

- Naturally or artificially fluoridated water supplies have been reported to reduce **dental caries** by as much as 50% to 70% and to reduce the incidence of osteoporosis as well.
- Prenatal fluoride improves fetal tooth development.
- 50 mg/d hardens remaining bone and prevents fractures in established **osteoporosis.**

Supplement Considerations

- Infant supplementation of 0.25 mg/d (1 mg/d for children and adults) is considered safe and adequate when other sources are absent.
- Circulating fluoride from diet or water is more effective than topical fluoride treatments or fluoride toothpastes.
- Supplements should be dissolved in the mouth if possible.
- Fluoride rinses once per week decrease tooth decay in school children by 20% to 40%.
- Toothpastes and rinses should not be swallowed.

Toxicity/Side Effects/Contraindications

- A fluoride concentration of 2 to 8 ppm in water has caused mottling, dulling, and pitting of teeth. Adequate calcium intake minimizes these effects.
- A concentration of more than 8 ppm in water as well as in some pharmaceutical doses have caused kidney dysfunction and arthritis-like symptoms.
- There is no evidence of increased cancer incidence from fluoridation.

GERMANIUM

- no established need in human nutrition

Occurrence

- unknown

US Dietary Intake

- unknown

Deficiency High-Risk or Increased-Need Groups

- unknown

Clinical Measurement

- no available tests

Deficiency Consequences

- unknown

Therapeutic Uses

- Claims for immune enhancement and antiviral and anticancer effects have not been formally studied in humans.
- Animal studies suggest immune stimulation and tumor inhibition.

Supplement Considerations

- Organic germanium 132 and germanium sesquioxide are available.

Toxicity/Side Effects/Contraindications

- Skin irritations and soft stools have been reported.
- There are some reports of contaminated supplements that caused kidney failure.

IODINE

- 1989 adult RDA = 150 μg/d

Occurrence

- iodized salt: 76 μg/g or 400 μg/tsp
- seafood: 50 to 150 μg per serving
- seaweed products: up to 4500 μg/g dry weight
- bread made with iodinated dough conditioners: up to 150 μg per slice
- dairy products: 50 to 100 μg per serving, depending on cattle feed content
- contained in Red No. 3.
- drinking water content highly variable

US Dietary Intake

- average intake—250 μg/d (adult male), and 170 μg/d (adult female) from food sources alone
- upper range of 5 to 10 times the RDA due to commercial use in bakery products, cattle feed, iodized salt, and food dye, as well as drinking water content

Deficiency High-Risk or Increased-Need Groups

- those with high intake of cabbage family and other foods containing natural goitrogens
- inhabitants of noncoastal regions if iodized salt not used

Clinical Measurement

- Urinary iodine/creatinine ratio reflects recent intake.
- Measures of thyroid function reflect availability of iodine for hormone synthesis if there is no hypothyroid condition from other causes.

Deficiency Consequences

- goiter, hypothyroidism
- cretinism in newborns

Therapeutic Uses

- Correction of dietary deficiency usually causes regression of goiter.
- 100 mg/d reduces thyroid uptake of radioactive iodide from nuclear power plant accidents. (Iodine should not be taken at this level for more than 1 to 2 weeks.)
- One report claimed relief from **fibrocystic breast disease** using large doses.

Supplement Considerations

- Supplementation is not recommended under normal circumstances.
- Saturated solutions of potassium iodide provide 30 mg per drop.

Toxicity/Side Effects/Contraindications

- Over 6 mg/d (40 times RDA) may affect thyroid function.
- Some individuals have a hypersensitivity reaction to iodine that causes rash, nausea, headache, and/or cough.
- Large amounts (over 1000 µg/d) are thought to aggravate acne.

IRON

- 1989 RDA = 10 mg/d adult male, 15 mg/d premenopausal adult female
- assumes omnivorous diet adequate in vitamin C

Occurrence and Availability

- 8 mg per serving—chicken liver
- 5 mg per serving—beef liver, oysters, crab, prunes, fortified cereals (poorer absorption)
- 3 mg per serving—beef, pork, turkey, dried fruit, blackstrap molasses
- 2 mg per serving—legumes, nuts, dark green vegetables
- 1 mg per serving—seafood, chicken, eggs, grains
- iron cookware (when used with acid foods)
- animal tissue sources containing heme iron better absorbed
- eggs and some plant sources contain absorption inhibitors
- vitamin C enhances absorption

US Dietary Intake

- males—17 mg/d average, 6.5 to 30 mg/d range; females—10.5 mg/d average, 4 to 20 mg/d range

- one third of all females considered deficient by RDA standards
- common US diet sources—meat, poultry, fish, eggs, fortified and enriched grain products

Deficiency High-Risk or Increased-Need Groups

- increased utilization: children up to age 4 years, adolescents, pregnant/multiparous females
- increased losses: menstruating females; those with frank or occult hemorrhage or surgery; those who use aspirin and other prostaglandin inhibitor drugs; endurance athletes
- decreased intake: weight loss dieters, vegetarians
- decreased absorption: elderly persons and vegetarians; those with malabsorption syndromes, low vitamin C intake, heavy use of tea/coffee/antacids, high dietary intake of oxalate/phosphate/phytate, chronic exposure to lead/cadmium

Clinical Measurement

- Serum iron reflects recent intake.
- Serum ferritin over 12 µg/L indicates adequate tissue stores.
- Anemia usually develops gradually after prolonged deficiency.
- Hair iron is not related to body iron levels.

Deficiency Consequences

- Microcytic hypochromic anemia affects 10% of US population.
- Early symptoms (may occur before anemia develops) include
  1. **fatigue**—muscle weakness, impaired work performance
  2. **impaired mental function**—learning disorders in children, behavior abnormalities in infants

3. decreased **cellular immunity**—more frequent/severe infections
- Incidence of deficiency: 5% to 14% of menstruating females, 4% to 12% of early adolescent males, 9% of children 1 to 2 years.

Therapeutic Uses

- Treatment of iron deficiency is the only known therapeutic use for iron.

Supplement Considerations

- Iron is available as sulfate, fumarate, gluconate, citrate, chelate, heme, and carbonyl.
- Heme iron is four or five times better absorbed; carbonyl iron is slightly better absorbed; other forms are equivalent to each other.
- Inorganic and nonheme forms are better absorbed in the presence of amino acids and vitamin C. Large doses are more poorly absorbed than small doses.
- Calcium carbonate and phosphate supplements inhibit absorption.
- 30 mg/d is recommended during pregnancy.
- 10 mg/d is recommended for infants and children.
- Supplements are recommended for most adults on low-calorie diets.

Toxicity/Side Effects/Contraindications

- Gastrointestinal distress may occur in sensitive individuals (take with meals) or when poorly absorbed.
- Inorganic iron destroys vitamin E on contact in the gastrointestinal tract—best to separate supplements.

- Iron is contraindicated in genetic hemachromatosis (high serum ferritin), which may afflict over 7% of population.
- Iron is contaidincated with tetracycline medication.
- Elderly patients with inflammatory and other chronic diseases may appear anemic and demonstrate low serum iron, yet may not be iron-deficient. Use serum ferritin to confirm true deficiency.
- Recent concern exists over whether iron excess causes free radical pathology. Large doses above daily requirements can lead to excessive accumulation in the body.

MAGNESIUM

- 1989 RDA = 4.5 mg/kg of body weight
- 1989 adult male RDA = 350 mg/d

Occurrence

- 75 mg per serving—spinach, chard
- 50 mg per serving—collards, eggplant, most legumes, nuts
- 25 mg per serving—milk, buttermilk, yogurt, lean red meats, poultry, seafood, whole-grain products, other green vegetables, corn, peas, squashes, sweet potatoes, grapefruit, melons
- all cheeses, seeds, lettuce and cabbage—low in magnesium

US Dietary Intake

- general range—200 to 500 mg/d
- adult males—329 mg/d average
- adult females—207 mg/d average
- approximately 120 mg/1000 kcal in average US diet, depending on food choices

Deficiency High-Risk or Increased-Need Groups

- alcohol abuse, chronic diarrhea, malabsorption syndromes
- some kidney diseases, use of some diuretics, digitalis therapy
- low-calorie diets, high coffee intake, laxative abuse
- heavy regular exercise, pregnancy
- older individuals, especially with high heart disease risk or diabetes

Clinical Measurement

- Serum levels reflect recent intake only.
- RBC or WBC magnesium correlate with tissue levels and more accurately indicate body status.
- Magnesium-loading tests measure urinary excretion after large doses. Low excretion rates suggest depleted body stores.
- Hair magnesium is less reliable; it may be high or low in deficient states and is always lower in gray hair.

Deficiency Consequences

- marginal levels associated with increased risk of cardiac arrhythmias, vasospastic angina, and fatal heart attacks
- muscle weakness, tremors, hypocalcemia, hypokalemia in advanced deficiency

Therapeutic Uses

- Intracellular imbalances of calcium and magnesium may be contributing factors in conditions such as
    1. **menstrual cramps,**
    2. **muscle cramps,**

3. **bronchial asthma**
4. **cardiac arrhythmia**
5. **coronary vasospasm**

- Intravenous magnesium reduced mortality in **heart attack** victims from 19% to 7%.
- 400 to 800 mg/d may reduce blood pressure in deficient **hypertensives.**
- 200 to 300 mg/d with 10 mg/d vitamin B6 helped prevent recurrent calcium oxalate **kidney stones.**
- 400 to 800 mg/d may help relieve symptoms of **premenstrual syndrome.**

Supplement Considerations

- Magnesium carbonate (in dolomite) is poorly absorbed.
- Magnesium oxide is concentrated but may be poorly absorbed if gastric acidity is deficient.
- Gluconate, aspartate, taurate, glycinate, and other chelated forms may be better absorbed, but are less concentrated.
- Intracellular concentration may be facilitated by additional vitamin B6.

Toxicity/Side Effects/Contraindications

- Magnesium is contraindicated in some individuals with impaired kidney function and in patients who have heart blocks without artificial pacemakers.
- Patients taking potassium-sparing diuretics or those with kidney dysfunction should be monitored for elevated serum magnesium during supplementation. Signs include hypotension, hyporeflexia, and depression of respiratory and cardiac function.
- Large doses of poorly absorbed forms may cause diarrhea.

MANGANESE

1989 adult ESADDI = 2.0 to 5.0 mg/d

Occurrence

- 1.0 to 1.5 mg per serving—whole-wheat products (phytates may reduce availability), nuts, pineapple, tea
- 0.60 to 0.75 mg per serving—wheat, rye, oat cereals
- 0.35 to 0.50 mg per serving—corn products, brown rice, berries, dark green leafy vegetables, legumes
- 0.15 to 0.25 mg per serving—white rice, bananas, dried fruit, enriched pasta, most nonstarchy vegetables

US Dietary Intake

- average adult intake—2.7 mg/d (male), and 2.2 mg/d (female)

Deficiency High-Risk or Increased-Need Groups

- high intakes of calcium, magnesium, iron, or phosphorus
- possibly intake of dietary factors antagonistic to any of the above minerals (phytate, tea, aluminum antacids, etc.)
- low blood levels in diabetes and pancreatic insufficiency
- low blood levels in patients with convulsive disorders and epilepsy
- low blood levels in osteoporotic women
- breast-fed infants usually in negative balance, although deficiency syndrome absent

Clinical Measurement

- No reliable normal values have been set for urinary or serum levels. Whole-blood or leukocyte manganese has been suggested as an indicator of tissue levels.
- Hair manganese is not a reliable measure of body levels; gray hair consistently shows lower concentrations.

Deficiency Consequences

- None is demonstrated in free-living humans; animals display developmental bone and joint defects, impaired reproductive function, and glucose intolerance.
- There is a possible increase in degenerative processes because of antioxidant role.
- Role in connective tissue synthesis suggests impaired musculoskeletal health and poor healing response to trauma, although this is based on animal studies only.

Therapeutic Uses

- 50 to 300 mg/d has been suggested for accelerating connective tissue repair in **trauma** and **degenerative joint disease.** No experimental evidence exists as yet that this is useful.

Supplement Considerations

- Manganese is very poorly absorbed (about 3% of dietary intake).
- Manganese is often supplied as manganese sulfate because of the requirement for sulfate in connective tissue synthesis.
- Manganese gluconate and chelate may be better absorbed.

Toxicity/Side Effects/Contraindications

- Low toxicity from oral ingestion unless absorption is enhanced by iron deficiency.
- High doses may partially block iron absorption.
- Nausea, gastrointestinal upset with doses of manganese sulfate over 100 mg/d have been reported.
- Chronic inhalation of manganese dust in mining and industrial sites has caused parkinsonian symptoms.

MOLYBDENUM

1989 adult ESADDI = 75 to 250 µg/d

Occurrence

- highest in dairy foods, legumes, organ meats, and grain products
- drinking water—2 to 8 µg/d

US Dietary Intake

- daily adult average—109 µg/d (male), 76 µg/d (female)

Deficiency High-Risk or Increased-Need Groups

- high intake of copper or sulfate/sulfite

Clinical Measurement

- detectable in hair trace mineral analysis, but significance unknown

Deficiency Consequences

- disturbed purine metabolism, reduced antioxidant protection
- increased sulfite sensitivity producing neurologic disturbances
- possible increased risk of esophageal cancer

Therapeutic Uses

- none proven at this time

Supplement Considerations

- Molybdenum is contained in some multivitamin/mineral products, usually as sodium molybdate.
- Consider concurrent copper supplementation.

Toxicity/Side Effects/Contraindications

- A dose of 540 µg/d has been associated with impaired copper status.
- High levels may increase incidence of gout.

PHOSPHORUS

- 1989 adult RDA = 800 mg/d
- 1989 young adult RDA = 1200 mg/d

Occurrence

- 250 mg per serving—milk, yogurt, buttermilk, milk puddings

- 200 mg per serving—meats, poultry, fish, processed cheeses (American, etc.), cottage cheese
- 100 mg per serving—eggs, unprocessed hard cheeses, bakery goods (in baking powder), legumes, nuts and seeds, avocado
- polyphosphate, phosphoric acid, and other absorbable additives are not usually counted in food tables

US Dietary Intake

- adult male average—1500 mg/d from natural sources
- adult female average—1000 mg/d from natural sources
- phosphate-containing food additives possibly contribute an additional 15% to 20% daily
- common sources—milk products, breads, beef products, eggs, alcoholic beverages
- average phosphorus/calcium ratio 1.5:1.0 but may be up to 4:1 for diets low in dairy products and green vegetables

Deficiency High-Risk or Increased-Need Groups

- deficiency very uncommon
- alcoholism, some kidney diseases, malabsorption syndromes
- possibly with chronic use of magnesium or aluminum hydroxide antacids, which bind phosphorus

Clinical Measurement

- Serum phosphorus does not vary with dietary intake.
- Urinary levels may reflect excessive intake.

Deficiency Consequences

- bone loss (osteomalacia)

Therapeutic Uses

- 4 grams/d for 6 days increased **endurance performance** in some athletes.

Supplement Considerations

- Phosphorus should not be present in most supplements because of abundance in US diet and possibility of adverse effects on calcium balance.
- Phosphate in mineral supplements inhibits absorption of iron and possibly other minerals.

Toxicity/Side Effects/Contraindications

- Phosphorus is contraindicated in kidney failure.
- Phosphorus/calcium ratio of 2:1 or greater is associated in some animals with bone resorption and soft tissue calcification. This may not be a problem in humans, however.
- Phosphorus as phytate in bran, whole grains, and legumes may inhibit mineral absorption if excessive.

POTASSIUM

- 1989 estimated minimum adult requirement = 2000 mg/d
- Desirable adult intake = approximately 3500 mg/d

Occurrence

- avocado—600 mg/half
- carrot juice—600 mg/8 oz
- cantaloupe—500 mg/cup
- dried fruit—500 mg per serving
- banana—450 mg each
- papaya—400 mg per half
- legumes—300 to 500 mg per serving
- milk products (not cheese)—400 mg per serving
- meat, poultry, seafood—200 to 400 mg per serving
- vegetables—200 to 300 mg per serving
- potatoes—300 to 500 mg per serving
- tomato sauce—400 mg per serving
- other fruits—100 to 300 mg per serving

US Dietary Intake

- adult males—typical range 1100 to 5500 mg/d (2900 average)
- adult females—typical range 700 to 4000 mg/d (2100 average)
- varies directly with amount of fruits and vegetables consumed—highest may reach 8 to 11 g/d

Deficiency High-Risk or Increased-Need Groups

- excessive diarrhea, vomiting or diuresis, Cushing's disease
- patients taking certain diuretics (thiazide or furosemide family, loop diuretics), corticosteroids, or cardiac drugs that are potassium-wasting
- high caffeine intake

Clinical Measurement

- 1 mEq potassium = 39 mg
- 1 mEq chloride = 35.5 mg
- 1 mmol potassium chloride = 74.5 mg
- potassium content of potassium chloride salt substitutes—52% by weight
- RBC potassium reflects tissue stores better than serum levels

Deficiency Consequences

- Early signs may include muscle weakness, bradycardia, and cardiac arrhythmia.
- Low intake is associated with higher risk of hypertension and stroke-related death.

Therapeutic Uses

- 4700 to 6800 mg/d total intake is associated with 3% to 10% drop in overall **blood pressure.** More dramatic effects are seen in African Americans. Supplemental potassium citrate or aspartate may be more effective than supplemental potassium chloride.
- Patients using potassium-wasting **diuretics** require approximately 1500 mg/d additional potassium.
- There is no indication that exercising athletes require potassium replacement.

Supplement Considerations

- Therapeutic doses required cannot be achieved easily with nonprescription supplements because of federal law restricting

potency to under 100 mg per tablet. Liquid supplements may circumvent this restriction.
- Commercial potassium salt substitutes provide approximately 2500 mg of potassium (60 to 70 mEq) per teaspoon. Seasoned salt substitutes provide approximately 1500 to 2000 milligrams (30 to 50 mEq) per teaspoon.

Toxicity/Side Effects/Contraindications

- Potassium is contraindicated in kidney failure and when potassium-sparing diuretics (spironolactone family, triampterene family) or angiotensin-converting enzyme inhibitors are taken.
- Elderly patients should be monitored for hyperkalemia.
- Potentially toxic doses usually cause nausea and vomiting, which prevents absorption.

SELENIUM

- 1989 adult RDA = 0.87 µg/kg of body weight
- 1989 adult male RDA = 70 µg/d

Occurrence

- up to ± 50% content depending on soil or feed content
- 100 µg per serving—tuna (limited bioavailability)
- 50 to 60 µg per serving—oysters, lobster, mussels, herring
- 35 to 50 µg per serving—ham
- 25 to 35 µg per serving—most fish, shrimp, poultry, beef
- 20 to 25 µg per serving—soft cheeses, lamb, pasta
- 10 to 15 µg per serving—hard cheeses, whole-grain products, luncheon meats

US Dietary Intake

- average adult intake—108 µg/d, range 62 to 224 µg/d
- soil in eastern and northwestern United States low in selenium (plants exposed to sulfur dioxide pollution or acid rain may take up less selenium as result)

Deficiency High-Risk or Increased-Need Groups

- alcohol abuse
- high cancer or heart disease risk (see below)
- exposure to ozone in smog pollution or toxic metals such as mercury and cadmium

Clinical Measurement

- Serum levels reflect recent intake.
- RBC selenium reflects tissue levels.
- Platelet or RBC glutathione peroxidase activity measures selenium need for optimal enzyme functioning.
- Hair selenium analysis has been validated, but it is difficult to measure and may be falsely elevated by use of selenium-containing shampoos.

Deficiency Consequences

- may cause excessive free-radical pathology because of reduced activity of selenium-dependent glutathione peroxidase enzyme
- increased risk of cancer of the colon, lung, breast, prostate, ovary, lymph glands, genitourinary tract, pancreas, and skin
- increased risk of cardiovascular disease, myocardial infarction, stroke, and heart disease mortality

- possible connections to all major degenerative diseases via increased free-radical pathology
- possible immune system suppression
- advanced deficiency causes muscle degeneration and cardiomyopathy

Therapeutic Uses

- Large doses with vitamin E have shown antitumor effects in animals with **breast cancer.**
- One study reported relief of **angina** symptoms using 1000 µg of selenium plus 200 IU of vitamin E.
- There is preliminary evidence of the usefulness of 400 to 1000 µg/d as an **immune system** stimulant.
- Selenium may be useful in the removal of **toxic heavy metals** from the body.
- Veterinary use of selenium/vitamin E combinations for arthritis has been reported, but no human studies have been done.

Supplement Considerations

- Some authorities have recommended 250 to 300 µg/d for cancer prevention.
- Selenium, especially organic forms, is relatively well absorbed compared with other minerals.
- Organic forms include selenomethionine, selenocysteine, amino acid chelates, yeast, and kelp-bound selenium. Selenocysteine is directly incorporated into glutathione peroxidase.
- Inorganic forms include selenite and selenate. Selenite may have greater antitumorigenic properties than organic forms. Vitamin C decreases the absorption of inorganic selenium.
- Selenium's action overlaps and is synergistic with that of vitamin E.

Toxicity/Side Effects/Contraindications

- Some authorities have proposed a maximal acceptable intake level of 500 μg/d.
- High water content of selenium in some areas has produced mild toxic effects.
- Intake of inorganic selenium of 1000 μg/d for prolonged periods has been reported to be toxic. Organic selenium does not produce this effect at this level.
- Toxicity signs include garlic breath odor, metallic taste in mouth, skin and nail changes, gastrointestinal irritation, dizziness.
- Moderate excesses may increase dental caries in children.

SILICON

- ESADDI unknown; 20 mg/d may be minimal need

Occurrence

- high in unrefined grain products, root vegetables

US Dietary Intake

- estimated at 21 to 46 mg/d

Deficiency High-Risk or Increased-Need Groups

- diets high in fiber, molybdenum, magnesium, or fluoride

Clinical Measurement

- detectable in hair trace mineral analysis, but significance unknown

Deficiency Consequences

- connective tissue and bone changes in animals

Therapeutic Uses

- speculation of usefulness in atherosclerosis, hypertension, and osteoarthritis

Supplement Considerations

- Horsetail (shave grass) herb contains significant amounts.

Toxicity/Side Effects/Contraindications

- Silicon has very low toxicity.
- Could possibly contribute to kidney stone formation in susceptible individuals.

SODIUM AND CHLORIDE

- 1989 estimated minimal adult requirement = 500 mg/d sodium, 750 mg/d chloride
- recommended maximal intake = 2400 mg/d sodium (6 g of salt)

Occurrence (in milligrams of sodium)

- salt—2300 mg/tsp
- lite salt—975 mg/tsp
- monosodium glutamate—615 mg/tsp
- soy sauce—200 to 345 mg/tsp
- ketchup, salad dressings—100 to 200 mg/Tbs
- gravies, most sauces—150 to 350 mg per serving (1/4 cup)
- tomato/spaghetti sauces—400 to 600 mg per serving (1/2 cup)
- fast-food hamburger—800 to 1600 mg
- pizza, cheese—1100 to 1400 mg per serving
- casseroles—800 to 1200 mg per serving
- burrito—650 to 1200 mg per serving
- Chinese food—700 to 1200 mg per serving
- fast food fried chicken—500 to 800 mg per serving
- ham—900 to 1300 mg per serving
- sausage, hot dogs—300 to 600 mg per serving
- luncheon meats, kosher meats—200 to 400 mg per serving
- smoked, cured, preserved, and pickled foods—300 to 700 mg per serving
- cheese and cheese products—200 to 350 mg per serving
- salty snack foods (chips, saltines, pretzels, etc.)—150 to 450 mg per serving
- commercial grain products, cereals, etc.—125 to 300 mg per serving
- canned vegetables—200 to 300 mg per serving
- seasoned vegetable dishes—400 to 600 mg per serving
- tomato/vegetable juice drinks—500 to 650 mg per serving
- canned soups—500 to 1000 mg per serving
- antacids containing sodium—500 to 1000 mg per tablet
- 1000 mg vitamin C as sodium ascorbate—130 mg
- chloride content of foods—usually 1.5 times sodium content

US Dietary Intake (Sodium)

- adult males—typical range 1100 to 8000 mg/d (3500 average) from food alone, average total salt intake 10 to 11 g/d
- adult females—typical range 700 to 5000 mg/d (2200 average) from food alone, average total salt intake from 5.5 to 10.3 g/d
- sources—75% from processed foods, 15% from salt added in cooking and at table, 10% from natural salt content of food (Breads, crackers, hot dogs, ham, luncheon meats, cheeses, soups, and tomato sauces make up one third of salt intake.)

Overingestion High-Risk or Restriction-Needed Groups

- hypertension (Approximately 75% of population develops elevated blood pressure by age 65 years; therefore most individuals should not overingest.)
- diuretic therapy
- heart failure with edema
- liver cirrhosis
- premenstrual bloating, idiopathic edema
- some evidence that chloride, not sodium, is offending component of salt

Clinical Measurement

- 1 mEq sodium = 23 mg
- 1 mEq chloride = 35.5 mg
- 1 (mmol) sodium chloride = 58.5 mg

Sodium content of salt is 39% by weight.
Serum levels are maintained independently of intake.
Twenty-four-hour urinary sodium reflects daily intake.

Low plasma renin activity following 3 days of sodium restriction helps identify hypertensives who will benefit from restriction.

Deficiency Consequences

- Deficiency is uncommon except in Addison's disease, some kidney diseases, extreme polyuria, or diarrhea.
- Excessive perspiration requires sodium replacement only after 8 lb or more of fluid are lost. This happens only after several hours of intense activity without sodium replacement. (See Chapter 25, "Sports Nutrition".)

Therapeutic Uses

- Restriction is important in heart failure and often in essential hypertension, especially if drug therapy is employed.
- Mild restriction (2 to 3 g/d sodium) is used for moderate heart failure and to enhance antihypertensive drug therapy; may reduce blood pressure by about 7/4 mm Hg without medication. Mild restriction would reduce stroke incidence by 26% and ischemic heart disease by 15% if adopted by Western populations, according to recent estimates.
- Moderate restriction (1 to 2 g/d sodium) is required for more severe hypertension; may reduce blood pressure in sodium-sensitive hypertensives about 14/7 mm Hg.
- Severe restriction (less than 1 g/d sodium) reliably lowers blood pressure in most hypertensives.

Supplement Considerations

- Use of salt tablets by athletes and factory workers is unnecessary and dangerous, and should be discouraged.

Micronutrients 329

- Electrolyte replacement beverages (sports drinks) should not contain large amounts (over 120 mg/8 oz) of sodium. Small amounts enhance rehydration.

Toxicity/Side Effects/Contraindications

- Sodium restriction is contraindicated in pregnancy-related hypertension.

VANADIUM

- ESADDI = 100 to 300 µg/d

Occurrence

- root vegetables, nuts, seafood, vegetable oils

US Dietary Intake

- estimated daily average—4 to 30 µg/d

Deficiency High-Risk or Increased-Need Groups

- unknown

Clinical Measurement

- detectable in hair trace mineral analysis, but significance unknown

Deficiency Consequences

- possible link to atherosclerosis

Therapeutic Uses

- preliminary evidence of insulinlike effects on glucose tolerance
- preliminary evidence of hypocholesterolemic effects

Supplement Considerations

- contained in some multivitamin/mineral products

Toxicity/Side Effects/Contraindications

- Increased levels have been suggested to be a factor in manic-depressive illness.
- Human equivalents of 200 µg/d have adversely affected some animals.

ZINC

- 1989 adult male RDA = 15 mg/d

Occurrence

- 20 mg each—oysters
- 2 to 3 mg per serving—beef, poultry, yogurt
- 1 mg per serving—most meats, poultry, seafood, dairy products, eggs, peanuts, whole grains

- 0.5 mg per serving—other legumes, whole-grain bread
- may not be as bioavailable in unleavened, unsprouted whole-grain products because of phytate content

US Dietary Intake

- 8.5 to 13 mg/d average range in most adults, 7 to 10 mg/d in elderly persons
- depends on protein intake; approximately 1.5 mg zinc per 10 g of protein in diet
- common sources—70% in US diet from animal products

Deficiency High-Risk or Increased-Need Groups

- inadequate intake: women during pregnancy and lactation, children from low-income families, elderly persons
- poor absorption: non-breast-fed infants; vegetarians using unleavened whole-grain products or bran; those with high iron, copper, or phosphorus intake; those with chronic exposure to mercury and cadmium; those with gastrointestinal disease; elderly persons, alcoholics
- increased utilization: those with severe trauma or infection, athletes, diabetics, those with sickle-cell anemia

Clinical Measurement

- Serum levels reflect recent intake.
- RBC or WBC zinc levels correlate with tissue levels.
- Hair zinc is less reliable, as it may be high or low in deficient states. Hair may also be contaminated by zinc-containing shampoos.
- The zinc taste test examines the ability to detect the bitter taste of a 0.1% solution of zinc sulfate. Correlation with other measures has not been adequately done as yet.

Deficiency Consequences

- growth retardation in children
- slow wound healing
- impaired taste, smell, and appetite
- decreased cell-mediated immunity
- impaired glucose tolerance, decreased alcohol tolerance
- increased oxidative tissue damage (free radical pathology)
- sterility in men, possibly impotence as well

Therapeutic Uses

- Zinc (30 to 150 mg/d) is the treatment of choice for **acrodermatitis enteropathica.**
- Zinc is an effective alternative to penicillamine in the treatment of Wilson's disease. See "Copper."
- 100 mg/d improved **immune function** in a group of healthy elderly persons.
- AIDS and many **cancer** patients often have reduced serum zinc levels.
- 90 to 150 mg/d has improved **pustular acne.**
- 150 mg/d improved healing rates for **gastric ulcers** and **surgical wounds.**
- 100 mg/d improved **rheumatoid arthritis** symptoms in one study but not in other, later, studies. **Psoriatic arthritis** also responded to zinc therapy in one study.
- Some, not all, studies suggested that a zinc lozenge supplement dissolved in the mouth may help cure **viral upper respiratory infections.** Doses every 2 hours are required up to a total of 150 to 300 mg/d for no more than 1 week.
- 200 mg/d reduced vision loss from **macular degeneration.**
- 50 mg/d may improve **sperm count** in men with **infertility.**
- Effectiveness in prostate disorders is theoretical only.

Supplement Considerations

- Zinc sulfate is not well tolerated by some persons (gastrointestinal irritation); taking with meals may improve tolerance.
- Zinc absorption is enhanced when taken with protein meals.
- Zinc citrate, aspartate, gluconate, and picolinate are better absorbed and rarely produce side effects.
- Zinc lozenges are indicated for local treatment of gastric ulcers and upper respiratory viral infections.
- Long-term high-dose zinc supplementation should include other trace elements, especially copper, to avoid deficiencies.

Toxicity/Side Effects/Contraindications

- Nausea, vomiting, diarrhea occur; required dose depends on type of zinc compound ingested (see above).
- Prolonged doses above 15 mg/d may impair copper and iron status.
- 50 to 150 mg/d without supplemental copper may lower HDL levels.
- 300 mg/d reduced lymphocyte responsiveness.

Bibliography for Part IV: Micronutrients

Alpers DH, Clouse RE, Stenson WF. *Manual of Nutrition Therapeutics.* Boston: Little, Brown and Co; 1988.

American Medical Association. *AMA Drug Evaluations.* Philadelphia: WB Saunders Co; 1983.

Austin S. *Clinical Nutrition* (seminar with bibliography). Portland, Ore: Western States Chiropractic College; 1991.

Austin S. *Clinical Nutrition Update* (periodical). Portland, Ore: Bergner Communications.

Bland JS. *Metabolic Update* (audio periodical with biblographies). Gig Harbor, Wash: HealthComm Inc; 1982–1985.

Brown ML, ed. *Present Knowledge in Nutrition.* 6th ed. Washington, DC: International Life Sciences Institute-Nutrition Foundation; 1990.

Buist R, ed. *International Clinical Nutrition Review* (periodical). Sydney, Australia: Integrated Therapies Pty Ltd.

Centers for Disease Control. *Ten-State Nutrition Survey, 1968–70.* Washington, DC: US Government Printing Office; 1972.

Consumer and Food Economics Institute. *Composition of Foods: Agriculture Handbooks No. 8-1 to 8-9.* Washington, DC: US Government Printing Office; 1976–1982.

Dickinson A. *Benefits of Nutritional Supplements.* Washington, DC: Council for Responsible Nutrition; 1987.

Dickinson A. *Safety of Vitamins and Minerals: A Summary of the Findings of Key Reviews.* Washington, DC: Council for Responsible Nutrition; 1986.

Food and Nutrition Board, National Research Council. *Recommended Dietary Allowances.* 10th ed. Washington, DC: National Academy Press; 1989.

Gaby AR, Wright JV. *Nutrition Therapy in Medical Practice* (seminar with bibliography). Los Angeles: Wright/Gaby Nutritional Seminars; 1985.

Hendler SS. *The Doctors' Vitamin and Mineral Encyclopedia.* New York: Simon and Schuster; 1990.

Krause MV, Mahan LK. *Food, Nutrition and Diet Therapy.* 7th ed. Philadelphia: WB Saunders Co; 1984.

Langseth L, ed. *Nutrition Research Newsletter* (periodical). Palisades, NY: Lyda Associates Inc.

Mckee G, ed. *Nutrition and the MD* (periodical). Los Angeles: PM Inc.

Monsen ER, ed. *Journal of the American Dietetic Association* (periodical). Chicago: American Dietetic Association.

Pennington J. *Food Values of Portions Commonly Used.* 15th ed. New York: Harper & Row; 1989.

Powers DE, Moore AO. *Food-Medication Interactions.* 6th ed. Tempe, Ariz: F-M-I Publ; 1988.

Shils ME, Young VR, eds. *Modern Nutrition in Health and Disease.* 7th ed. Philadelphia: Lea & Febiger; 1988.

Werbach MR. *Nutritional Influences on Illness: A Sourcebook of Clinical Research.* Tarzana, Calif: Third Line Press; 1988.

Werbach MR. *Nutritional Influences on Mental Illness: A Sourcebook of Clinical Research.* Tarzana, Calif: Third Line Press; 1991.

Williams SR. *Nutrition and Diet Therapy.* St. Louis, Mo: CV Mosby Co; 1989.

Appendices

Appendix A. Prostaglandins and Related Eicosanoids

I. Eicosanoid functions
   A. Inflammatory/anti-inflammatory
      1. Implicated in arthritis, dermatitis, mastitis
   B. Smooth muscle contraction/relaxation
      1. Implicated in hypertension, asthma, dysmenorrhea
   C. Promote/inhibit platelet aggregation
      1. Implicated in thrombotic disease, atherosclerosis, myocardial infarction
   D. Regulate immune function
II. Eicosanoid structure and nomenclature
   A. Usually 20 carbons in length
   B. 5-member ring in center
      1. Various modifications of ring possible
   C. Three major groups
      1. PG—prostaglandins
      2. TX—thromboxanes
      3. LT—leukotrienes
   D. Ring modifications
      1. A, B, C, D, E, F, G, H, I, depending on modification
   E. Number of double bonds
      1. 1, 2, 3, 4 in subscript
   F. Common examples—PGE_1, PGE_2, PGF_2, PGI_2, TXA_2, LTA_4, LTB_4
III. Eicosanoid precursors: omega-6 (ω-6) and omega-3 (ω-3) fatty acids
   A. Dihomo γ-linolenic acid (DGLA)—C20:3 ω-6

1. Produced in liver by desaturation and elongation of linoleic acid (LA)—C18:2 ω-6
    a. Found in most vegetable oils
    b. Desaturation requires zinc, vitamin B6, and magnesium
2. Naturally occurring (7% to 24%) in evening primrose, black currant, and borage oils
3. Precursor to 1-series PG and TX, which are generally benign
B. Arachidonic acid—C20:4 ω-6
    1. Produced in liver by desaturation of DGLA
        a. Inhibited by eicosapentaenoic acid (EPA)
    2. Naturally occurring in flesh foods, dairy fat, and shellfish
    3. Precursor to 2-series PG, TX, and 4-series LT, which are implicated in many pathologic conditions
C. Eicosapentaenoic acid (EPA)—C20:5 ω-3 and docosahexaenoic acid (DHA)—C22:6 ω-3
    1. Naturally occurring in seafood
    2. Produced inefficiently in human liver by desaturation and elongation of α-linolenic acid (ALA)—C18:3 ω-3
        a. ALA found in linseed (flaxseed) oil, soy oil, walnut oil, wheat germ oil
        b. Desaturation requires zinc, vitamin B6, and magnesium; inhibited by alcohol and *trans* fatty acids
    3. Precursor to 3-series PG, TX, and 5-series LT, which are generally weakly active
IV. Eicosanoid synthesis
    A. Precursors are available in cell membrane phospholipids OR as serum free fatty acids, cholesterol esters, and phospholipids.
    B. Phospholipid-bound fatty acids must be released by phospholipase A_2 enzyme before it can be used for PG, TX, or LT synthesis.
        1. Corticosteroid hormones and vitamin E inhibit this enzyme.

Appendix A: Prostaglandins and Related Eicosanoids 341

- C. Cyclo-oxygenase is the chief enzyme for PG and TX synthesis.
    1. Aspirin and nonsteroidal anti-inflammatory drugs inhibit this enzyme.
    2. Vitamin E inhibits this enzyme.
    3. Most long-chain unsaturated fatty acids compete for this enzyme.
- D. Lipo-oxygenase is the chief enzyme for LT synthesis.
    1. Inhibited by some experimental drugs, vitamin E, and certain bioflavonoids.
    2. Most long-chain unsaturated fatty acids compete for this enzyme.

V. Nutritional and pharmacologic manipulation
- A. Excess arachidonic acid metabolites may be significant in the pathophysiology of diseases associated with prostaglandin imblance.
    1. Prostaglandin 2-series
    2. Thromboxane 2-series
    3. Leukotriene 4-series
- B. Therapeutic intervention using the following dietary modifications and supplements may minimize the production of the above metabolites as follows.
    1. Minimize dietary sources of arachidonic acid.
        a. Limit flesh foods, dairy, shellfish.
    2. Minimize endogenous synthesis of arachidonic acid.
        a. Increase dietary/supplemental EPA.
    3. Minimize availability of arachidonic acid in membrane and circulating lipids.
        a. Increase dietary/supplemental linoleic acid, linolenic acid, DGLA, and/or EPA.
    4. Minimize release of arachidonic acid following pathologic stimuli.
        a. High-dose vitamin E (400+ IU/d).
    5. Minimize enzymatic conversion of arachidonic acid to its metabolites.

a. Aspirin and nonsteroidal anti-inflammatory drugs
   b. Competition from LA, ALA, DGLA, and EPA
   c. High-dose vitamin E (400+ IU/d)
   d. High-dose bioflavonoids (1000 to 2000 mg/d)
C. At the same time, synthesis of benign 1-series and 3-series prostaglandins should be unimpeded.
   1. Ensure adequate intake of vitamin B6, magnesium, and zinc.
   2. Avoid *trans* fatty acids and alcohol.

Appendix B. Free Radicals and Lipid Peroxidation

I. Definition of free radicals
   A. Molecular fragment with unpaired electron
   B. Highly reactive and short-lived
   C. Oxygen radicals most common in human biochemistry
II. Occurrence
   A. Nonpathologic examples
      1. Lysosomal action of phagocytic leukocytes
      2. Hepatic cytochrome P-450 reactions
      3. Mitochondrial processes
      4. Many oxidative enzyme reactions
   B. Pathologic examples
      1. X-ray damage
      2. Toxicity of various herbicides and pesticides
      3. Aging processes (controversial)
      4. Degenerative disease (controversial)
         a. Linked with autoimmune disorders, cancer, atherosclerosis, liver disease
III. Production and fate of oxygen radicals
   A. Superoxide from molecular oxygen
      1. Less toxic than other free radicals.
      2. Dismutates spontaneously or in presence of superoxide dismutase enzyme to form hydrogen peroxide.
      3. May contribute to the production of more highly toxic hydroxyl radical.
   B. Singlet oxygen from molecular oxygen
      1. Not strictly a free radical; one member of electron pair is excited to a higher orbital.

2. Formation requires ionizing energy source (ultraviolet) or chemical excitation.
C. Hydroxyl radical from hydrogen peroxide (in presence of superoxide and iron or copper)
   1. Extremely toxic
   2. Can attack unsaturated fatty acids in living systems to produce lipid radicals
D. Lipid peroxyl radicals and hydroperoxides from polyunsaturated fatty acids (lipid peroxidation)
   1. Occurs in living systems, not in foods.
   2. Initial formation requires hydroxyl radical.
      a. Lipid peroxyl radicals can chain-react with nearby lipids to form additional radicals and hydroperoxides.
      b. Lipid hydroperoxides can react with iron to form additional radicals.

IV. Toxic effects of oxygen radicals and intermediates
   A. Cell membrane damage through lipid peroxidation by hydroxyl and lipid peroxyl radicals
   B. DNA damage by hydroxyl radical, superoxide radical, or singlet oxygen

V. Cellular defenses against oxygen radicals
   A. Enzymatic
      1. Superoxide dismutase—two forms
         a. Contains zinc/copper or manganese.
         b. Produces hydrogen peroxide.
      2. Catalase
         a. Reduces hydrogen peroxide to water and oxygen.
      3. Glutathione peroxidase
         a. Contains selenium.
         b. Requires glutathione and glutathione reductase.
         c. Reduces hydrogen peroxide to oxygen and water.
         d. Reduces lipid hydroperoxides to lipid alcohols and water.
   B. Non-enzymatic (antioxidants)

Appendix B: Free Radicals and Lipid Peroxidation 345

1. Vitamin E
   a. Neutralizes lipid radicals and possibly singlet oxygen.
   b. Interrupts lipid radical chain reactions.
2. Beta carotene
   a. Neutralizes singlet oxygen, possibly other free radicals.
3. Vitamin C
   a. Neutralizes free radicals in aqueous compartments.
   b. Helps regenerate vitamin E.
4. Glutathione
   a. Cofactor for glutathione peroxidase.
   b. May neutralize some free radicals directly.
   c. Helps regenerate vitamin E.

Appendix C. Carbohydrate Biochemistry and Physiology

I. General characteristics
   A. Complex carbohydrates—polysaccharides normally associated with fiber
      1. Amylose—straight-chain glucose polymer found in plant starch (grains, legumes, roots, tubers, gourds, etc.)
      2. Amylopectin—branched-chain glucose polymer also found in plant starch
      3. Glycogen—animal starch, does not significantly contribute to dietary carbohydrate (1% of muscle tissue by weight)
   B. Simple sugars—monosaccharides and disaccharides
      1. Sucrose—dimer of glucose and fructose, which is found naturally in certain foods but largely used as an added sweetener
      2. Lactose—dimer of glucose and galactose found only in milk products
      3. Fructose (levulose)—monomer found in fruits, corn syrup sweeteners, and dietetic foods; 1.7 times sweeter than sucrose; US intake is increasing dramatically
      4. Glucose (dextrose) and other sugars—found in free form primarily in fruits and some vegetables
      5. Corn syrup is mostly glucose unless converted enzymatically to high-fructose form
      6. Invert sugar and honey are both mixtures of glucose and fructose
      7. Maple sugar is mostly sucrose

Appendix C: Carbohydrate Biochemistry and Physiology 347

   8. Fruits are from 3% (melon) to 64% (fig) sugar and may contain glucose, fructose, sucrose, or combinations of these.
C. Sugar substitutes—used as non-nutritive and/or noncariogenic alternatives to sugar
   1. Saccharin—synthetic, suspected carcinogen
   2. Cyclamate—synthetic, suspected carcinogen
   3. Aspartame—synthetic, health risks controversial
   4. Acesulfame-K—synthetic, undergoing safety testing prior to approval
   5. Mannitol, Sorbitol—naturally occurring, nutritive, noncariogenic, possible diarrhea in large amounts
   6. Xylitol—naturally occurring, nutritive, noncariogenic, possible diarrhea, possible carcinogen
D. Dietary fiber—usually composed of carbohydrates, but does not contribute much to caloric intake because of its low digestibility.
   1. Structural categories
      a. Cellulose (insoluble)—a straight-chain glucose polymer (β-1,4 linkage) found in the cell wall of plants.
      b. Hemicellulose (soluble and insoluble)—a branched-chain polymer of various sugars and sugar derivatives found in the plant cell wall.
      c. Pectin (soluble)—a polymer of galacturonic acid used by plants as intercellular cement.
      d. Algin (soluble)—a polymer of various sugar derivatives used in the cell walls of algae and seaweed.
      e. Gums and mucilages (soluble)—various polymers of sugar derivatives found in plant sap and other secretions.
      f. Lignin (insoluble)—not a polysaccharide, but an aromatic hydrocarbon chain found in the cell wall of woody plant parts.
      g. "Crude" fiber is an antiquated term that referred only to the insoluble fibers.

2. Common characteristics
   a. They are hydrophilic, ie, they retain water.
   b. Soluble fibers form gels.
   c. Some can bind metallic ions and other substances (bile acids for example).
   d. Many can be broken down by intestinal bacteria, releasing absorbable end-products.
3. Water-insoluble fibers exert mechanical effects on the intestinal tract.
   a. They increase fecal bulk, which stimulates peristalsis and reduces intraluminal pressure.
4. Water-soluble fibers exert systemic as well as mechanical effects that may influence the whole body.
   a. They "normalize" transit time.
   b. They form gels that lubricate the fecal bolus.
   c. They form a mechanical barrier to absorption of nutrients (desirable for excessive dietary fat and sugar).
   d. They bind toxic metal contaminants of food.
   e. Some may bind bile acids, preventing their recirculation to the liver and forcing conversion of additional cholesterol.
   f. Some are partially digested, and their end-products may be absorbed and affect cholesterol metabolism.

II. Overview of carbohydrate digestion and absorption
   A. Mouth—salivary amylase
      1. Begins breaking primary starch linkages, producing maltose and dextrins.
      2. Inactivated by stomach pH.
   B. Duodenum—pancreatic amylase
      1. Requires alkaline pH.
      2. Continues hydrolysis of primary starch linkages.
      3. Reduces 95% of polysaccharides to molecules of six or fewer monosaccharide units.
   C. Intestinal brush border—several enzymes

Appendix C: Carbohydrate Biochemistry and Physiology 349

      1. Maltase—breaks primary glucose-glucose bonds.
      2. Dextrinase—breaks glucose-glucose bonds at branching points.
      3. Sucrase—breaks glucose-fructose bond.
      4. Lactase—breaks glucose-galactose bond.
   D. Only monosaccharides are absorbed from the gut lumen in appreciable amounts.
   E. Some dietary fiber is broken down and metabolized into absorbable fatty acids by colonic bacteria.
III. Regulation of blood sugar levels (Figure C-1)
   A. Glucose, representing about 70% of absorbed sugars, must be removed from the blood into the tissues where it will be used.

Figure C-1 Normal glucose tolerance curve

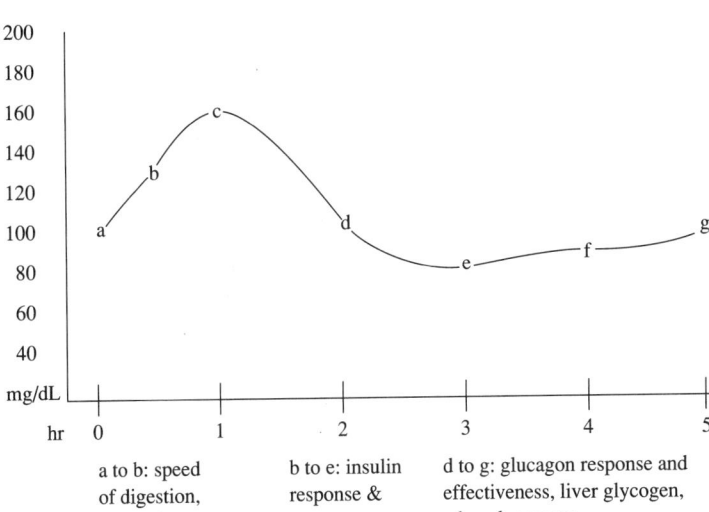

1. Blood glucose levels must be maintained within normal limits of about 65 to 115 mg/dL.
2. The average meal causes blood glucose to rise about 25 to 50 mg/dL, returning to normal within 2 to 3 hours.
3. The ability of a carbohydrate-containing food to raise and maintain elevated blood sugar during the first 2 hours after it is eaten has been designated the **glycemic index** for that food.
4. The glycemic index depends on speed of glucose entry into circulation before adequate visceral and hormonal response is possible. Factors affecting this speed are:
    a. amount of glucose present in food (versus other monosaccharides)
    b. rate of food ingestion (effect of liquids, concentration)
    c. rate of gastric emptying (effect of fat, soluble fiber)
    d. ability of digestive enzymes to interact efficiently with food carbohydrate (physical form, chemical or mechanical inhibitors)
    e. amount of digestion required to produce free glucose (effect of chain length food processing, cooking)
    f. degree of glucose intolerance of the individual (effect of genetics, pathology, physical fitness, nutrition)

B. Glucose diffuses freely into two major tissues.
  1. Liver—which, under the influence of insulin, can handle glucose in three ways.
     a. Catabolize it to produce ATP for hepatocellular use.
     b. Store it as glycogen.
     c. Convert it to triglyceride and either store it or send it back into the general circulation on very-low-density lipoproteins.
  2. Brain—highly dependent on glucose for energy and an important site of glucose consumption in the body.

C. Glucose requires the presence of insulin to gain entry into the other major tissues, notably adipose and muscle.

Appendix C: Carbohydrate Biochemistry and Physiology 351

1. The pancreas is stimulated to produce insulin by two mechanisms.
   a. Increase in blood glucose concentration
   b. Presence of sugar (glucose or sucrose) and other foodstuffs in small intestine, which stimulates release of a gastric hormone (gastric inhibitory peptide) that promotes insulin secretion
2. Normal insulin production requires certain nutrients.
   a. Protein for polypeptide synthesis
   b. Zinc for storage and activation of prohormone
3. Insulin reduces blood glucose levels by binding to cell membrane receptors, thus stimulating active transport of glucose into cells.
4. A second factor, produced in the liver, appears to facilitate the effects of insulin on peripheral tissues.
   a. Called **glucose tolerance factor** (GTF), its structure appears to include chromium, niacin, and three amino acids—glutamic acid, glycine, and cysteine.
   b. In some individuals who demonstrate a lowered ability to bind insulin to cells (obese, diabetic), supplemental chromium has been shown to increase insulin binding.
5. Insulin also affects the metabolism of glucose in three ways.
   a. Increases production of ATP from glucose.
   b. Increases production of glycogen from glucose.
   c. Increases triglyceride synthesis from glucose.

D. The effects of insulin are balanced by the actions of other hormones.
   1. Glucagon from the pancreas causes glycogenolysis and gluconeogenesis in the liver.
      a. Gluconeogenesis can use most amino acids, glycerol from fat, and some organic acids as precursors for glucose.
   2. Epinephrine and norepinephrine from the adrenal medulla causes glycogenolysis in the liver, muscle tissue, and heart and gluconeogenesis in the liver.

3. Glucocorticoids from the adrenal cortex cause gluconeogenesis in the liver.
4. Growth hormone from the anterior pituitary causes glycogenolysis in the liver, increased blood insulin levels, and increased insulin resistance in the peripheral tissues.

E. Long-term blood sugar maintenance
1. Hepatic glycogenolysis peaks 8 hours into fasting and is normally depleted within 24 to 28 hours.
2. Hepatic and eventually renal gluconeogenesis peaks after 24 hours of fasting and can function indefinitely.

IV. Carbohydrates as an energy source
A. Glycogenolysis releases glucose from glycogen stores in liver and all types of muscle.
 1. Liver glycogen may replenish blood glucose and therefore supply energy to all tissues.
 2. Muscle glycogen can be utilized only by the cell in which it is stored.
B. Glycolysis produces pyruvate and some high-energy electrons from glucose.
 1. Requires niacin, phosphate, and magnesium.
C. Oxidative decarboxylation of pyruvate produces acetyl-coenzyme A and some high-energy electrons.
 1. Requires thiamine, riboflavin, niacin, pantothenic acid, and magnesium.
D. Citric acid (Krebs') cycle oxidizes acetyl-coenzyme A to produce more high-energy electrons.
 1. Requires thiamine, riboflavin, niacin, biotin, and magnesium.
E. Electron transport chain transfers energy from the high-energy electrons to molecules of ATP.
 1. Requires riboflavin, niacin, iron, sulfur, copper, and magnesium.

V. Carbohydrates and connective tissue
A. Connective tissue structure

Appendix C: Carbohydrate Biochemistry and Physiology 353

      1. Fibrous proteins provide structural strength, especially in tendons, ligaments, annular fibers, etc.
         a. Includes collagen, elastin, and keratin
      2. Proteoglycans (glycosaminoglycans, or mucopolysaccharides) provide shock absorption and lubrication, especially in cartilage, bone matrix, joint fluid, nucleus pulposis, etc.
         a. Includes chondroitin sulfates and hyaluronic acid.
         b. Synthesized by chondrocytes.
    B. Proteoglycan structure and synthesis
      1. Derived sugars—hexosamines and hexuronic acids—are linked together into:
         a. Carbohydrate "coils," dozens of which are attached to a strand of protein by:
         b. Glycosyltransferase enzyme
            (1) Requires manganese as an essential cofactor
      2. Sulfation of the coils increases bulk and compressibility
VI. Other functions of carbohydrates
    A. Prevent excessive use of protein for energy needs
    B. Prevent excessive ketone production from overutilization of fats for energy
    C. Other specialized molecules
      1. Glucuronic acid used in liver detoxification mechanisms, conjugation of bilirubin, estrogen, etc.
      2. Ribose required for nucleic acid synthesis
      3. Glycoproteins function as antibodies, cell receptors, blood clotting factors, etc.
      4. Glycolipids function in neural tissue

Appendix D. Lipid Biochemistry and Physiology

I. Classification
   A. Simple lipids contain water-insoluble molecules made of carbon, hydrogen, and (often) oxygen.
      1. Fatty acids are long-chain carboxylic acids (see II for examples).
      2. Triglycerides are esters of one glycerol molecule and three fatty acids.
      3. Other fatty acid esters use very complex alcohols such as sterols (cholesterol ester) or certain vitamins (retinyl palmitate, tocopherol acetate).
   B. Compound lipids contain simple lipids combined with nonlipid molecules.
      1. Phosphoglycerides contain phosphoric acid and alcohol substituted onto the terminal carbon of triglycerides.
         a. Example—lecithin, containing choline, functions in cell membrane structure, fat transport, and fat utilization.
      2. Sphingolipids are derivatives of sphingosine containing phosphate, organic amines, or carbohydrate.
         a. Sphingomyelins, containing phosphate and choline, are found in cell membrane of many tissues.
         b. Cerebrosides and gangliosides have special functions in nerve tissue and elsewhere.
      3. Lipoproteins, containing triglyceride, cholesterol, lecithin, and protein, are all involved in fat transport in the blood (see "Transport/lipoprotein metabolism" below).

Appendix D: Lipid Biochemistry and Physiology 355

      a. Chylomicrons
      b. Very-low-density lipoprotein (VLDL)
      c. Low-density lipoprotein (LDL)
      d. High-density lipoprotein (HDL)
  C. Sterols are complex alcohols with multiple-ring structures.
    1. Cholesterol is essential to cell membrane and myelin structure and is an important precursor in biosynthesis of other steroids.
    2. Steroid hormones are produced in the adrenals and the gonads.
    3. Vitamin D, after conversion to active vitamin D hormone, has effects on calcium metabolism.
II. Fatty acid nomenclature
  A. Four characteristics are required to describe structure.
    1. Carbon chain length (C16, C18, C20, etc.)
    2. Degree of unsaturation (:0, :1, :2, :3, etc.)
    3. Location of double bonds (ω-3, ω-6, ω-9)
    4. Stereochemistry (*cis, trans*)
  B. Common examples in clinical nutrition:
    1. Stearic acid (C18:0)
    2. Oleic acid (*cis* C18:1 ω-9)
    3. Linoleic acid (*cis* C18:2 ω-6)
    4. γ-linolenic acid (*cis* C18:3 ω-6)
    5. Arachidonic acid (*cis* C20:4 ω-6)
    6. α-linolenic acid (*cis* C18:3 ω-3)
    7. Eicosapentaenoic acid (*cis* C20:5 ω-3)
    8. Docosahexaenoic acid (*cis* C22:6 ω-3)
III. Digestion/absorption
  A. Bile emulsification forms smaller lipid droplets having greater total surface area for enzymes to attack.
  B. Pancreatic secretions provide digestive enzymes.
    1. Lipase cleaves fatty acids from triglycerides.
    2. Phospholipase cleaves fatty acids from phospholipids.
    3. Cholesterol esterase removes fatty acids from cholesterol ester to produce free cholesterol.

C. Micelle formation via interaction of bile salt and fat digestion byproducts facilitates absorption into intestinal cells.
IV. Transport/lipoprotein metabolism
   A. Chylomicron formation, function, and metabolism
      1. Fat digestion byproducts are resynthesized by the intestinal cell into triglycerides, phospholipids, and cholesterol ester.
      2. Chylomicrons are formed from the absorbed resynthesized fats plus apoprotein B-48, which influences chylomicron metabolism.
      3. Chylomicrons are transported by the intestinal lacteal vessels to the subclavian vein.
      4. In the circulation, chylomicrons receive apoproteins C-2 and E from high-density liproprotein (HDL).
      5. In the capillaries, apoprotein C-2 activates lipoprotein lipase, which removes triglyceride from the chylomicrons, allowing fatty acids to be taken up by tissue cells.
      6. As the chylomicrons are depleted of triglyceride, apoprotein C-2 is returned to HDL.
      7. The chylomicron remnants are recognized by liver cell receptors by virtue of their apoproteins B-48 and E and are taken into the liver.
   B. Very-low-density lipoprotein (VLDL) formation, function, and metabolism
      1. The liver receives dietary cholesterol, phospholipid, and fat-soluble vitamins from chylomicron remnants.
      2. The liver synthesizes triglyceride from excess dietary sugars and other molecules and synthesizes cholesterol as well.
      3. The liver forms VLDL from the above fats plus apoprotein B-100 and releases VLDL into circulation.
      4. In the circulation, VLDL receives apoproteins C-2 and E from HDL.
      5. In the capillaries, apoprotein C-2 activates lipoprotein lipase, which removes triglyceride from VLDL, allowing tissue cells to uptake triglyceride.

Appendix D: Lipid Biochemistry and Physiology 357

  6. As VLDL is depleted of triglyceride, apoproteins C-2 and E are returned to HDL along with phospholipid and free cholesterol, while cholesterol ester is simultaneously transferred from HDL to VLDL.
      a. This exchange reaction is accomplished in the circulation by cholesterol ester transfer protein located on HDL.
  7. The above modifications cause VLDL to be gradually transformed to intermediate-density lipoprotein (IDL) and then to low-density lipoprotein (LDL).
C. LDL function and metabolism
  1. LDL contains primarily free cholesterol and cholesterol ester, along with certain fat-soluble vitamins and apoprotein B-100.
  2. LDL is small enough to escape circulation into the extracellular spaces of peripheral tissues, where it delivers cholesterol to cells.
  3. Tissue cell receptors recognize apoprotein B-100 and uptake LDL into the cell by endocytosis.
  4. LDL is degraded by intracellular enzymes, releasing cholesterol and other substances for use by the cell.
  5. As cells accumulate LDL cholesterol, they (ideally) reduce their own cholesterol synthesis and reduce the number of membrane LDL receptors.
D. HDL formation, function, and metabolism
  1. HDL is produced in the liver and secreted into the circulation to interact with other lipoproteins (see above) and to scavenge excess tissue cholesterol and return it to the liver.
  2. HDL receives free cholesterol both from cell membrane surfaces and from other lipoproteins in circulation.
  3. Free cholesterol in HDL is esterified by the enzyme phosphatidylcholine:cholesterol acyl transferase (PCAT, also known as LCAT where L = lecithin).

4. HDL-esterified cholesterol can be transferred to VLDL or LDL via cholesterol ester transfer protein, or the entire HDL particle may be taken up by the liver.
5. As the liver accumulates cholesterol, it can (ideally) reduce its own cholesterol synthesis, re-export cholesterol on VLDL, utilize cholesterol in the synthesis of bile acids, or secrete it directly into the digestive tract via the bile.

V. Fat as energy source
   A. Metabolic demand for fat
      1. Low after a meal, so fat tends to be stored.
      2. High during fasting or prolonged exercise, so fat tends to be mobilized.
   B. Hormonal influences on lipolysis
      1. Triglyceride in fat cells is broken down and fatty acids are released when insulin levels are low and either glucagon or epinephrine levels are high.
   C. Catabolism of fatty acids
      1. Free fatty acid transport in serum
         a. Fatty acids from lipolysis are transported on serum albumin to the tissues (exceptions—cannot be utilized by nervous system or RBCs).
      2. Intracellular transport mechanisms
         a. Fatty acids are transported into mitochondria by carnitine.
      3. β-Oxidation produces acetyl-coenzyme A from fatty acids.
         a. Requires riboflavin, niacin, biotin, vitamin B12
      4. Acetyl-coenzyme A may enter tricarboxylic acid (Krebs') cycle or, in liver, may be converted to ketones.

VI. Fatty acids and prostaglandins—see Appendix A.

VII. Lipid peroxidation—see Appendix B.

Appendix E. Protein Biochemistry and Physiology

I. Protein contributions
   A. Nitrogen in the form of amino groups for synthesis of nonessential amino acids and other nitrogen compounds
   B. Essential amino acids and, under certain conditions, other amino acids that may not always be synthesized in sufficient quantities
      1. Essential: histidine, lysine, leucine, isoleucine, valine, threonine, methionine, phenylalanine, tryptophan
      2. Conditionally essential: arginine (infants), tyrosine (prematurity, phenylketonuria), taurine, carnitine (genetic defects or specific pathology), etc.
   C. Energy is derived from certain amounts of protein in the diet.
II. Protein requirements
   A. Depends on protein quality
      1. Amino acid balance—some amino acids are required in greater amounts than others.
         a. Animal proteins most resemble human amino acid patterns and are highly concentrated and digestible.
         b. Plant proteins eaten as part of a mixed diet contribute very effectively to the body's amino acid pool.
      2. Digestibility—how much is absorbed
         a. Appears related to fiber content of a meal
   B. Factors that increase requirements
      1. Higher growth rates
      2. Lower efficiency of amino acid synthesis and conservation, as in certain diseases

3. Lower calorie intake
4. Lower protein quality

III. Digestion/absorption
   A. Gastric hydrocholoric acid and pepsin—accomplish less than 10% of protein digestion.
   B. Pancreatic proteases—digest dietary and endogenous protein.
      1. Endogenous protein (sloughed-off gut cells and enzymes) may account for up to 50% of digestion load.
   C. Intestinal peptidases—reduce particles to free amino acids, dipeptides, and tripeptides.
   D. Intestinal transport mechanisms
      1. Numerous pathways exist for different amino acids and small peptides.
      2. Small quantities of intact proteins can be absorbed as well.

IV. Amino acid metabolism
   A. The small intestine reduces small peptides to free amino acids and utilizes a large amount for its own protein synthesis.
      1. Proteins of the small intestine are turned over once in less than 1 day.
   B. Seventy-five percent of amino acids released into portal circulation are taken up by the liver.
      1. Some undergo intrahepatic conversion to other amino acids.
      2. Some are incorporated into proteins (plasma proteins, etc.).
      3. Some are deaminated and used for energy.
   C. The remaining amino acids are taken up by tissue cells.
      1. All cells synthesize protein from these amino acids (enzymes, structural proteins, etc.).
      2. Specialized tissues produce unique proteins.
         a. Plasma cells—immunoglobulins
         b. Pancreas—insulin, glucagon, digestive enzymes
         c. Bone marrow—hemoglobin
         d. Connective tissue—collagen, elastin, etc.
         e. Muscle—myoglobin, actin, myosin

Appendix E: Protein Biochemistry and Physiology 361

       3. Muscle cells also utilize a large amount of the branched-chain amino acids (valine, leucine, isoleucine) for energy.
- V. Hormone influences
  - A. Growth hormone—increases protein synthesis in all tissues.
  - B. Testosterone—increases protein synthesis primarily in muscle tissue.
  - C. Insulin—increases amino acid transport (especially branched-chain and aromatic amino acids) into muscle.
  - D. Corticosteroids—increases protein breakdown in muscle, bone, etc.
  - E. Thyroid hormone—variable depending on hormone level, calorie intake, and available amino acids.
- VI. Specific amino acid products
  - A. Neurotransmitters from tryptophan, tyrosine, glutamate, etc.
  - B. Thyroid hormone from tyrosine
  - C. Choline from serine and methionine
  - D. Vitamin B3 from tryptophan
  - E. Nucleic acids from aspartate, glutamine, and glycine
  - F. Bile acid conjugates from glycine and taurine
  - G. Heme from glycine
  - H. Creatine from methionine, glycine, and arginine
- VII. Amino acid and nitrogen catabolism
  - A. Excess amino acids are degraded in the liver.
    1. Yields keto acids, which must be utilized in anabolic processes or oxidized as energy sources.
    2. Yields ammonia, which is converted to urea and excreted.
  - B. Creatine, used in muscle energy metabolism, is regularly turned over to yield creatinine, which is excreted.
  - C. Nucleic acids contain nitrogen-laden purines and pyrimidines, which are regularly turned over.
    1. Pyrimidines are catabolized to carbon dioxide and ammonia.
       a. Requires vitamin B12.
    2. Purines are converted to uric acid, which is excreted.

Appendix F. Vitamin Biochemistry and Physiology

FAT-SOLUBLE VITAMINS

I. General characteristics
   A. Structural similarities, not functional ones.
   B. Absorption requires sufficient bile and pancreatic secretions.
   C. Packaged into chylomicrons for uptake by lymph circulation, which carries them to general circulation.
   D. Stored in various body tissues.
   E. Normally not excreted in urine.
II. Vitamin A
   A. Animal forms—retinol, retinal, retinoic acid
      1. Occurs naturally as fatty acid retinyl esters.
   B. Provitamin from plants—beta carotene and other carotenoids
   C. Absorption/transport/storage/excretion
      1. Retinyl esters (70% to 90%) absorbed after removal of fatty acid in intestine.
      2. Carotenes (20% to 60%) absorbed intact, then inefficiently split into retinal in gut cell.
      3. Absorption and utilization enhanced by dietary fat, protein, and vitamin E.
      4. Absorption decreased by oxidized fats and other oxidizing agents; deficiencies of protein; excess vitamin E, iron, and zinc.
      5. Vitamin A products then re-esterified for transport along with unconverted carotene in chylomicrons.

Appendix F: Vitamin Biochemistry and Physiology 363

      6. Total body vitamin A (90%) stored in liver.
      7. Retinol transported to tissues on retinol-binding protein and transthyretin.
      8. Carotenes distributed widely to adipose, adrenals, and other tissues.
      9. Excreted retinol first inactivated by liver, then eliminated in bile or urine.
    D. Functions
      1. Assists vision via rhodopsin (retinene) synthesis.
      2. Cell differentiation and maintenence
      3. Growth of bone, mucopolysaccharide synthesis
      4. Immune function and resistance to infection
      5. Influences iron metabolism.
    E. Carotenes have antioxidant activity superior to that of retinoids.
III. Vitamin D
    A. Natural form—cholecalciferol (vitamin D3)
    B. Alternate form—ergocalciferol (vitamin D2)
    C. Biosynthesis
      1. 7-dehydrocholesterol converted to vitamin D3 in skin cell via sunlight (affected by latitude, skin pigmentation, sunscreen).
      2. Vitamin D hydroxylated in liver to 25-hydroxyvitamin D3 (two to five times more potent than vitamin D).
      3. Second hydroxylation in kidney produces 1,25 dihydroxyvitamin D3 (calcitriol, active Vitamin D hormone, 10 times more potent than vitamin D).
      4. Calcitriol synthesis is regulated by parathyroid hormone and serum phosphate levels.
      5. Final conversion in kidney may be impaired with aging.
    D. Absorption/transport/storage/excretion
      1. Ingested vitamin D absorbed with other fats.
      2. Vitamin D from skin or gut transported on vitamin D plasma-binding protein to liver or other tissues for storage.

3. Excreted in bile after deactivation by the liver.
E. Functions
1. Gastrointestinal absorption of calcium and phosphate via synthesis of binding proteins
2. With parathyroid hormone, maintains serum calcium and phosphate by mobilization of bone stores.
3. Vitamin D receptors in other tissues have been identified, with unknown significance.

IV. Vitamin E
A. Eight natural isomers
1. d-α-Tocopherol (RRR-α-tocopherol) is the most potent form.
2. Other forms are β-, δ-, and γ-tocopherol and the four tocotrienols.
B. One major synthetic form
1. dl-α-tocopherol acetate (all-rac-α-tocopherol).
C. Relative to the potency of d-α-tocopherol (100%), the potencies of other significant forms are as follows:
1. d-α-tocopherol acetate 91%
2. dl-α-tocopherol acetate 74%
3. d-β-tocopherol 50%
4. d-γ-tocopherol 10%
5. d-α-tocotrienol 30%
D. When only d-α content is known, the contribution of other tocopherols in foods or supplements (mixed tocopherols) is about 20% additional vitamin E activity.
E. Susceptible to freezing.
F. Absorption/transport/storage/excretion
1. Absorption along with other dietary fats is 20% to 80%; with higher doses the percentage of absorption decreases.
2. Transported via chylomicrons to liver, which exports vitamin E on VLDL. Transferred to LDL and HDL in blood stream, which deliver vitamin E to cells.

3. Associated with cell membrane phospholipids in all cells. Larger amounts stored in fatty tissue.
G. Adult deficiency appears very slowly, only after 5 to 10 years of malabsorption, for example.
H. Functions
   1. Biologic antioxidant; prevents lipid peroxidation, especially important in cell membrane phospholipids that are highly polyunsaturated.
      a. Higher dietary polyunsaturated fat intake increases need for vitamin E.
      b. At least 0.6 IU of vitamin E required per gram of dietary polyunsaturated fat.

V. Vitamin K
   A. Nomenclature
      1. Plant form—phylloquinone (vitamin K1)
      2. Bacterial form—menaquinone (vitamin K2)
      3. Synthetic form—menadione (vitamin K3)
   B. Intestinal bacteria normally provide large amounts in humans, although not enough to prevent deficiencies.
   C. Absorption/transport/storage/excretion
      1. Absorption along with other dietary fats is 40% to 70% in small intestine, much less in colon.
      2. Transported via chylomicrons to liver, where small amounts are stored.
      3. Distributed on other lipoproteins to many body tissues, where it usually concentrates in intracellular membranes.
      4. Excreted in bile and urine.
   D. Functions
      1. Prothrombin synthesis via carboxylation of glutamate, synthesis of other blood-clotting factors
      2. Osteocalcin synthesis (for calcium binding in bone and kidney)

WATER-SOLUBLE VITAMINS

VI. Vitamin B1
   A. Nomenclature
      1. In diet: thiamine
      2. Coenzyme form: thiamine pyrophosphate (TPP)
   B. Absorption/transport/storage/excretion
      1. Easily absorbed unless large amounts of alcohol or raw fish (containing microbes with thiaminase enzyme) are ingested.
      2. Most is phosphorylated to active form in the intestinal cells.
      3. Wide distribution to all tissues.
   C. Functions
      1. Coenzyme for oxidative decarboxylation reactions
         a. Pyruvate decarboxylase (producing acetyl-coenzyme A for Krebs' cycle, synthesis of lipids, acetylcholine, etc.)
         b. Lipid synthesis
      2. Other dehydrogenase complexes
      3. Coenzyme for transketolase enzyme in pentose phosphate pathway
      4. Additional role in nerve cell activity (poorly understood)
VII. Vitamin B2
   A. Nomenclature
      1. In diet: riboflavin.
      2. Coenzyme forms: riboflavin-5-phosphate (flavin mononucleotide, or FMN) or flavin adenine dinucleotide (FAD).
   B. Absorption/transport/storage/excretion
      1. Easily absorbed up to a 25-mg dose from intestine after cleavage of any phosphate groups by digestive enzymes.
      2. Phosphorylated in many tissues to FMN, and then a large amount is further converted to FAD.

Appendix F: Vitamin Biochemistry and Physiology 367

   3. Excreted in many metabolized forms in urine.
      a. Appears as a yellowish fluorescent pigment.
   C. Functions
      1. Contained in two coenzymes—FAD and FMN.
      2. These coenzymes can donate electrons singly or in pairs, catalyzing many oxidation-reduction reactions.
         a. Catabolism of carbohydrate and fatty acids
         b. Electron transport in mitochondria
         c. Metabolism of vitamins B3 and B6
         d. Certain antioxidant mechanisms (glutathione reductase)
VIII. Vitamin B3
   A. Nomenclature
      1. Plant source—niacin (nicotinic acid)
      2. Animal source—niacinamide (nicotinamide)
      3. Coenzyme forms—nicotinamide adenine dinucleotide (NAD) and nicotinamide adenine dinucleotide phosphate (NADP)
   B. Absorption/transport/storage/excretion
      1. Easily absorbed from the stomach and intestine.
      2. Converted to coenzymes in various tissues.
      3. Tryptophan converted to NAD in the liver.
         a. Sixty milligrams dietary tryptophan is equivalent to one milligram niacin.
      4. Very little storage; metabolites are excreted in the urine.
   C. Functions
      1. Two coenzymes
         a. NAD catalyzes many catabolic oxidation-reduction reactions such as glycolysis, tricarboxylic acid (Krebs') cycle, electron transport, etc.
         b. NADP catalyzes many anabolic oxidation-reduction reactions such as fatty acid synthesis, cholesterol synthesis, pentose shunt.
      2. Niacin idiosyncrasies

            a. In large doses initially produces rapid vasodilation of cutaneous blood vessels by prostaglandin-mediated stimulation of histamine release.
            b. Large doses lower serum cholesterol and triglyceride levels by several mechanisms, including inhibition of VLDL secretion by the liver.
            c. (Niacinamide has none of these effects.)
IX. Vitamin B5
    A. Nomenclature
        1. In diet: pantothenic acid
        2. In cellular metabolism: part of coenzyme A and acyl carrier protein
    B. Absorption/transport/storage/excretion
        1. Dietary coenzyme A is broken down by intestinal enzymes to release panthothenate, which is easily absorbed and transported to all tissues.
        2. Not stored
        3. Excreted in urine
    C. Functions
        1. Coenzyme A acts as a carrier molecule in acetylation (two-carbon) and acylation (multiple carbon) reactions:
            a. Energy metabolism
            b. Synthesis of acetylcholine, cholesterol, steroid hormones, porphyrin for heme synthesis, etc.
X. Vitamin B6
    A. Nomenclature
        1. In diet: pyridoxine, also pyridoxal, pyridoxamine
        2. In cellular metabolism: mostly pyridoxal-5-phosphate
    B. Requirement depends on dietary protein intake.
        1. 1.6 mg B6 for every 100 g dietary protein in healthy individuals
    C. Susceptible to freezing
    D. Absorption/transport/storage/excretion

1. All three forms are easily absorbed from the upper small intestine after cleavage of any phosphate groups by digestive enzymes.
2. Phosphorylation and oxidation to coenzyme forms occur in the intestinal cells after absorption and in other cells.
3. Transported either as free vitamin or as coenzyme attached to albumin and concentrated especially in muscle tissue.
4. Metabolites excreted in the urine.

E. Functions
1. Coenzyme in many reactions of amino acid metabolism—transamination, deamination, desulfuration, decarboxylation.
2. Also required for synthesis of heme, myelin, and neurotransmitters; production of prostaglandins; and release of stored glycogen in liver and muscle.

XI. Folic acid
A. Nomenclature
1. In diet: pteroylglutamic acid and pteroylpolyglutamic acid
2. In cellular metabolism: tetrahydrofolic acid
B. Sensitive to heat
C. Absorption/transport/storage/excretion
1. Dietary folic acid must have polyglutamate portion cleaved to monoglutamate in the intestine by intestinal enzymes (50% or less efficiency).
2. Monoglutamate form is absorbed in upper small intestine by active transport (50 to 90% absorption).
    a. Supplemental folic acid is better absorbed than most of dietary folate.
3. Converted to active forms in intestinal cells and elsewhere.
4. Three to six months' supply stored in liver and other tissues.
5. Various forms excreted in bile and urine.

D. Functions
  1. Single-carbon (methyl, formyl, etc.) transfer in synthesis and metabolism of purines, pyrimidines, amino acids, choline, heme, etc.
  2. Role in nucleic acid synthesis is important for the maturation of blood cells and other rapidly dividing tissues.

XII. Vitamin B12
  A. Nomenclature
    1. In diet: cobalamin (cyanocobalamin in supplements)
    2. Active forms: methylcobalamin, coenzyme B12
  B. Biologic sources
    1. Synthesized by bacteria, fungi, and yeasts only.
    2. Food sources must accumulate vitamin B12 from these organisms.
    3. Some synthesis by small intestinal bacteria may occur.
  C. Absorption/transport/storage/excretion
    1. Dietary amounts of vitamin B12 are released from food proteins by action of gastric HCl and proteases.
    2. In the alkaline intestine, it binds to intrinsic factor secreted from gastric parietal cells.
    3. Seventy percent of dietary quantities absorbed at specific receptor sites in terminal ileum.
    4. Pharmacologic doses may achieve 1% to 3% absorption by simple diffusion without intrinsic factor.
    5. Some evidence for nasal but not sublingual absorption.
    6. Transported via transcobalamin II protein in serum to cells.
    7. Two to three years' supply stored primarily in the liver.
    8. Excreted primarily in bile, which allows recirculation if intrinsic factor is present.
  D. Functions
    1. Regeneration of active folic acid for nucleic acid synthesis
    2. Coenzyme in fatty acid, amino acid, and thymine degradation
    3. Essential for normal myelin synthesis

Appendix F: Vitamin Biochemistry and Physiology 371

XIII. Biotin
   A. Synthesized by intestinal microorganisms
   B. Absorption/transport/storage/excretion
      1. Readily absorbed from dietary biotin, biotin-containing enzymes in food, and bacterial biotin.
      2. Avidin, found in raw egg white, prevents biotin absorption in large amounts.
      3. Not stored.
      4. Excreted in urine.
   C. Functions
      1. Coenzyme for carboxylation reactions
         a. Fatty acid synthesis, gluconeogenesis, energy metabolism, amino acid metabolism

XIV. Vitamin C
   A. Nomenclature
      1. In diet: mostly L-ascorbic acid.
      2. L-Ascorbic acid may be reversibly converted to L-dehydroascorbic acid (redox couple).
   B. Most unstable vitamin.
   C. Absorption/transport/storage/excretion
      1. Efficient absorption at dietary levels; absorption drops to as low as 50% with megadoses.
      2. Serum levels plateau when dietary intake reaches 90 to 150 mg/d; tissues are saturated at intakes above 200 mg/d.
      3. Highest tissue concentrations in leukocytes, adrenals.
      4. Total body capacity is no higher than 3000 mg.
      5. Oxalate is main urinary excretion product (up to 100 mg/d).
         a. Higher intake causes excretion of unchanged ascorbate in urine as well as bacterial degradation in intestine.
      6. Normal body stores are depleted gradually at about 3% loss per day if no vitamin C is ingested.
   D. Functions
      1. Collagen synthesis via hydroxylation of proline and lysine

2. Hormone and neurotransmitter synthesis (steroids, catecholamines, serotonin)
3. Bile acid synthesis (from cholesterol)
4. Antioxidant in water-soluble compartments
5. Immune function effector
6. Facilitates inorganic iron absorption

Appendix G. Mineral Biochemistry and Physiology

MACROMINERALS

I. Calcium
   A. Most abundant mineral in human body
   B. Absorption/transport/storage/excretion
      1. 30% to 50% of dietary calcium absorbed in nonelderly humans, usually less from large supplemental doses, more in deficiency states.
         a. Absorption facilitated by vitamin D-induced calcium-binding protein in intestinal cell.
      2. Transported in serum mostly as free ion and protein-bound calcium with small amounts complexed with citrate, sulfate, or phosphate.
      3. Serum levels regulated by parathormone, calcitonin, and calcitriol through action on bone, kidney, and intestine.
      4. Accumulated in bone primarily during growth with an additional 5% to 10% storage up to 10 years after longitudinal growth ceases.
         a. Present in bone as calcium phosphate [$Ca_3(PO_4)_2$] and hydroxyapatite [$Ca_{10}(PO_4)_6(OH)_6$].
      5. Over 99% of body calcium is concentrated in bones and teeth.
      6. Dietary excesses and tissue losses excreted in urine.
      7. Aging-related bone loss begins around 40 to 45 years of age.

a. Up to 0.5% bone loss per year in men and women, except for 2% to 5% loss per year for about 10 years after menopause in women not receiving hormone and mineral replacement.
C. Functions
1. Component of hydroxyapatite in bone.
2. Cofactor in blood clotting, cell membrane transport, muscle contraction, and heartbeat.
3. Intracellular second messenger for actions of neurotransmitters, enzymes, hormones, etc.

II. Phosphorus
A. Ubiquitous in nature, primarily as phosphate (PO_4) ion
B. Wide variety of metabolic functions
C. Absorption/transport/storage/excretion
1. Dietary phosphate well absorbed at 70% to 80%.
2. Serum transport as phosphoric acid buffers and protein-bound phosphate.
3. Constant calcium/phosphorus ratio is hormonally maintained in blood.
4. Stored in bone as calcium phosphate [$Ca_3(PO_4)_2$] and hydroxyapatite [$Ca_{10}(PO_4)_6(OH)_6$].
5. Over 85% concentrated in bones and teeth.
6. Excreted in the urine, although a large capacity for tubular reabsorption exists in deficiency states.
D. Functions
1. Forms high-energy phosphate linkages with adenosine, creatine, glucose, etc.
2. Essential component of phospholipids, nucleic acids, and hydroxyapatite.
3. Acid-base buffer component, especially inside cells.
4. Used in control mechanisms that regulate some enzyme activities (eg, phosphorylase).

III. Sulfur
A. Occurs in methionine, cysteine, taurine.

Appendix G: Mineral Biochemistry and Physiology 375

   B. Occurs in thiamine, biotin, coenzyme A, and acyl carrier protein.
   C. Absorption/transport/storage/excretion
      1. Absorbed and metabolized as sulfur amino acids.
      2. Excreted as sulfate in urine after amino acid catabolism.
   D. Functions
      1. Component of most proteins.
         a. Determines special characteristics of certain proteins such as collagen, keratins, insulin.
      2. Component of glutathione, a cellular antioxidant and amino acid transport cofactor.

IV. Magnesium
   A. Absorption/transport/storage/excretion
      1. Dietary levels absorbed from 25% to 70%.
         a. Absorption decreased at high intake levels and with high calcium or phosphate intake.
      2. Serum transport as free ion, protein-bound, and complexed with citrate, phosphate, etc.
      3. Concentrated intracellularly.
      4. Over 65% concentrated in storage sites in bone and over 25% concentrated in all muscle tissues.
      5. Excreted in the urine, although a large capacity for tubular reabsorption exists in deficiency states.
   B. Functions
      1. Cofactor in reactions involving high-energy phosphate compounds in energy metabolism and protein synthesis.
      2. Interacts in a poorly understood manner with calcium in neuromuscular transmission.
      3. Structural component of bone.

V. Fluoride
   A. Absorption/transport/storage/excretion
      1. Absorbed from the stomach and intestine at 50% to 80% efficiency.
      2. Serum transport as free ion and hydrogen fluoride.

3. Concentrated almost completely in bone and teeth, although uptake decreases with age.
4. Excreted in urine.

B. Functions
1. Replaces hydroxyl group of hydroxyapatite in bones and teeth, increasing resistance to demineralization and possibly inhibiting plaque bacteria.

VI. Electrolytes
A. Distribution
1. Sodium—extracellular cation
2. Chloride—extracellular anion (along with bicarbonate)
3. Potassium—intracellular cation (along with phosphate)

B. Absorption/transport/storage/excretion
1. Completely absorbed in upper small intestine.
2. Electrolyte balance strenuously regulated by mineralocorticoids (aldosterone), renin-angiotensin, and sympathetic nervous system.
3. Excreted in urine.

C. Functions
1. Water balance between body and environment.
2. Osmotic balance between membranes.
3. Acid-base balance along with bicarbonate ion.
4. Neuromuscular excitability.
5. Potassium is used in the regulation of enzyme activity.

VII. Iron
A. Occurs in nature as heme iron (surrounded by porphyrin ring) and nonheme iron.
B. Absorption/transport/storage/excretion
1. Wide range of intestinal absorption (less than 1% to more than 50%), which varies with body needs.
2. Absorption of nonheme iron enhanced by adequate stomach acid and either ascorbic acid or flesh foods.
3. Absorption decreased by tea, coffee, phosphates, phytate.
4. Transported on transferrin protein.

Appendix G: Mineral Biochemistry and Physiology 377

5. Stored as ferritin or hemosiderin in spleen, liver, and bone marrow.
6. 90% is conserved and reutilized from degradation of heme, enzymes, etc.
7. Excreted primarily in feces, menstrual fluid, and skin.

C. Functions
   1. Oxygen transport as hemoglobin in blood and oxygen storage as myoglobin in muscle
   2. Cofactor in cellular respiration (electron-transport system) as component of cytochromes, iron-sulfur proteins, and iron-containing flavoproteins
   3. Component of some antioxidant enzymes
   4. Important in cellular immunity and carnitine synthesis

TRACE MINERALS

I. Boron
   A. Absorption/transport/storage/excretion
      1. Boron, sodium borate, and boric acid are readily absorbed and excreted in the urine.
      2. More highly concentrated in bone than other tissues.
   B. Functions
      1. Affects macromineral (calcium, phosphorus, magnesium, potassium) metabolism, possibly through effects on metabolism of estrogen or other steroid hormones.

II. Chromium
   A. Absorption/transport/storage/excretion
      1. 0.5% to 2% absorption of trivalent (+3) chromium in food and supplements
         a. Absorption facilitated by amino acids; serum transport on transferrin or albumin.
      2. Concentrated in liver as glucose tolerance factor and in hair

3. Urinary excretion only
   a. Increased by excessive dietary sugars.
B. Functions
   1. Component of glucose tolerance factor (along with niacin and certain amino acids), which potentiates effect of insulin.
   2. May help regulate serum cholesterol and triglycerides.
   3. May activate several other enzymes.

III. Copper
   A. Absorption/transport/storage/excretion
      1. Absorption, primarily from duodenum, is 25% to 60%.
         a. Absorption enhanced by phytate(!).
         b. Absorption impaired by high intake of zinc, ascorbic acid, and possibly fructose.
      2. Excess uptake bound to metallothioneine in intestinal cell and secreted back into lumen.
      3. After albumin transport to liver, serum transport is mostly as ceruloplasmin, which donates copper to tissues.
      4. Stored in liver as metallothioneine.
      5. Excreted primarily in feces through biliary secretion.
   B. Functions
      1. Cofactor in oxidase enzymes—cytochrome oxidase, tyrosinase, dopamine hydroxylase, etc.
      2. Important for iron transport.
      3. Cofactor in connective tissue metabolism, including bone and vascular connective tissue.
      4. Plays a role in central nervous system structure and function.
      5. Component (with zinc) of cytoplasmic superoxide dismutase.

IV. Iodine
   A. Absorption/transport/storage/excretion
      1. Easily absorbed as iodide ion.
      2. Serum transport as free ion and protein-bound.
      3. Stored in thyroid gland.

4. Thyroid hormone degradation yields recyclable iodine.
5. Excreted in urine.
B. Functions
 1. Constituent of thyroxine (T_4—4 iodines) and triiodotyrosine (T_3—3 iodines), which regulate the rate of cellular metabolism.

V. Manganese
 A. Absorption/transport/storage/excretion
  1. Poorly absorbed (about 3%) from intestinal tract.
  2. Serum transport on transmanganin protein.
  3. Concentrated in mitochondria.
  4. Excreted in feces following biliary secretion.
 B. Functions
  1. Cofactor in synthesis of chondroitin sulfate and other mucopolysaccharide components of connective tissue.
  2. Cofactor for pyruvate carboxylase in carbohydrate metabolism, superoxide dismutase in mitochondria, and arginase in urea cycle.

VI. Molybdenum
 A. Absorption/transport/storage/excretion
  1. Between 25% and 80% absorbed as molybdate (MoO_4^{2-}) ion in stomach and intestine.
  2. Transported loosely attached to erythrocytes.
  3. Concentrated in liver, bone, and kidney.
  4. Excreted in urine and bile.
 B. Functions
  1. Component of xanthine oxidase in uric acid synthesis, sulfite oxidase in sulfur metabolism, and aldehyde oxidase in liver detoxification systems.

VII. Nickel
 A. Absorption/transport/storage/excretion
  1. Less than 10% of food nickel, but up to 50% nickel in water is absorbed.
  2. Serum transport mainly on albumin.

3. Widely distributed in tissues.
4. Excreted in urine.
B. Functions
1. May stabilize tertiary structure of nucleic acids and proteins.
2. Enhances absorption of ferric iron.
3. Possible enzyme cofactor.

VIII. Silicon
A. Absorption/transport/storage/excretion
1. Absorbed and transported as silicic acid $(Si(OH)_4)$.
2. Concentrated in connective tissue and skin.
3. Excreted in urine.
B. Functions
1. Participates in synthesis and structure of connective tissue and in the initiation of bone calcification.

IX. Selenium
A. Exists in nature primarily as selenocysteine (animal) and selenomethionine (plant), in which it replaces the sulfur atoms of those amino acids.
B. Absorption/transport/storage/excretion
1. Dietary and supplemental absorption is very efficient (>50%).
2. Transported on albumin or other proteins.
3. Dietary selenocysteine is degraded to anionic selenium, which then is utilized by tissues to resynthesize selenocysteine.
4. Dietary selenomethionine is not metabolically active, but becomes a storage pool for replacing selenium in deficiency states.
5. Excreted in urine.
B. Functions
1. Component, as selenocysteine, of glutathione peroxidase, which prevents accumulation of lipid and water-soluble peroxides that may contribute to cellular oxidative damage.

Appendix G: Mineral Biochemistry and Physiology 381

    2. Synergistic with antioxidant effect of vitamin E.
X. Vanadium
    A. Absorption/transport/storage/excretion
        1. Less than 5% absorbed.
        2. Several dietary forms exist, but serum transport is on transferrin and ferritin as vanadyl (VO^{2+}) ion.
        3. Concentrated in bone and liver.
        4. Excreted in urine.
    B. Functions
        1. May help regulate high-energy phosphate transfer enzymes.
        2. Many other unconfirmed roles have been suggested.
XI. Zinc
    A. Absorption/transport/storage/excretion
        1. Dietary zinc absorbed at less than 40%, with wide variation depending on body needs and many other factors.
        2. Absorption enhanced by histidine, glutathione, picolinate, and citrate.
        3. Absorption impaired by pancreatic dysfunction and high intakes of phytate, oxalate, phosphate, calcium, iron, or copper.
        4. Excess uptake bound to metallothioneine in gut cell and secreted back into lumen.
        5. Transported on albumin first to liver, then redistributed to other tissues.
        6. Concentrated in muscle, bone, and blood cells.
        7. Excreted primarily in feces.
    B. Functions
        1. Component of over 70 metalloenzymes
        2. Most important in nucleic acid and protein synthesis and metabolism
        3. Also important in immune function and cell membrane function
        4. Cofactor in carbonic anhydrase, alkaline phosphatase,

lactic acid dehydrogenase, carboxypeptidase, and cytoplasmic superoxide dismutase
5. Complexed with insulin in pancreatic beta cells

Bibliography for Appendices A–G

Brown ML, ed. *Present Knowledge in Nutrition*. 6th ed. Washington, DC: International Life Sciences Institute-Nutrition Foundation; 1990.

Champe PC, Harvey RA. *Lippincott's Illustrated Reviews: Biochemistry*. Philadelphia: JB Lippincott Co; 1987.

Dormandy TL. An approach to free radicals. *Lancet*. 1983;2:1010–1014.

Dormandy TL. Free-radical pathology and medicine: a review. *J R Coll Physicians Lond*. 1989;23:221–227.

Ganong WF. *Medical Physiology*. 13th ed. Norwalk, Conn: Appleton & Lange; 1987.

Lindner MC. *Nutritional Biochemistry and Metabolism with Clinical Applications*. New York: Elsevier Scientific Publishers; 1985.

Murray RK, Granner DK, Mayes PA, Rodwell VW. *Harper's Biochemistry*. 21st ed. Norwalk, Conn: Appleton & Lange; 1988.

Newsholme EA, Leech AR. *Biochemistry for the Medical Sciences*. New York: John Wiley & Sons; 1983.

Shils ME, Young VR, eds. *Modern Nutrition in Health and Disease*. Philadelphia: Lea & Febiger; 1988.

Willis AL. Nutritional and pharmacological factors in eicosanoid biology. *Nutr Rev*. 1981;39:289–301.

Appendix H. 1989 Recommended Dietary Allowances

FOOD AND NUTRITION BOARD, NATIONAL
RECOMMENDED DIETARY
Designed for the maintenance of good nutrition

Category	Age (years) or Condition	Weight[b] (kg)	Weight[b] (lb)	Height[b] (cm)	Height[b] (in)	Protein (g)	Fat-Soluble Vitamins			
							Vitamin A (μg RE)[c]	Vitamin D (μg)[d]	Vitamin E (mg α-TE)[e]	Vitamin K (μg)
Infants	0.0–0.5	6	13	60	24	13	375	7.5	3	5
	0.5–1.0	9	20	71	28	14	375	10	4	10
Children	1–3	13	29	90	35	16	400	10	6	15
	4–6	20	44	112	44	24	500	10	7	20
	7–10	28	62	132	52	28	700	10	7	30
Males	11–14	45	99	157	62	45	1,000	10	10	45
	15–18	66	145	176	69	59	1,000	10	10	65
	19–24	72	160	177	70	58	1,000	10	10	70
	25–50	79	174	176	70	63	1,000	5	10	80
	51+	77	170	173	68	63	1,000	5	10	80
Females	11–14	46	101	157	62	46	800	10	8	45
	15–18	55	120	163	64	44	800	10	8	55
	19–24	58	128	164	65	46	800	10	8	60
	25–50	63	138	163	64	50	800	5	8	65
	51+	65	143	160	63	50	800	5	8	65
Pregnant						60	800	10	10	65
Lactating	1st 6 months					65	1,300	10	12	65
	2nd 6 months					62	1,200	10	11	65

[a]The allowances, expressed as average daily intakes over time, are intended to provide for individual variations among most normal persons as they live in the United States under usual environmental stresses. Diets should be based on a variety of common foods in order to provide other nutrients for which human requirements have been less well defined.

[b]Weights and heights of Reference Adults are actual medians for the U.S. population of the designated age, as reported by NHANES II. The median weights and heights of those under 19 years of age were taken from Hamill et al. (1979) (see pages 16–17). The use of these figures does not imply that the height-to-weight ratios are ideal.

Appendix H: 1989 Recommended Dietary Allowances

ACADEMY OF SCIENCES—NATIONAL RESEARCH COUNCIL
ALLOWANCES,[a] Revised 1989
of practically all healthy people in the United States

Water-Soluble Vitamins							Minerals							
Vitamin C (mg)	Thiamin (mg)	Riboflavin (mg)	Niacin (mg NE)[f]	Vitamin B_6 (mg)	Folate (μg)	Vitamin B_{12} (μg)	Calcium (mg)	Phosphorus (mg)	Magnesium (mg)	Iron (mg)	Zinc (mg)	Iodine (μg)	Selenium (μg)
30	0.3	0.4	5	0.3	25	0.3	400	300	40	6	5	40	10
35	0.4	0.5	6	0.6	35	0.5	600	500	60	10	5	50	15
40	0.7	0.8	9	1.0	50	0.7	800	800	80	10	10	70	20
45	0.9	1.1	12	1.1	75	1.0	800	800	120	10	10	90	20
45	1.0	1.2	13	1.4	100	1.4	800	800	170	10	10	120	30
50	1.3	1.5	17	1.7	150	2.0	1,200	1,200	270	12	15	150	40
60	1.5	1.8	20	2.0	200	2.0	1,200	1,200	400	12	15	150	50
60	1.5	1.7	19	2.0	200	2.0	1,200	1,200	350	10	15	150	70
60	1.5	1.7	19	2.0	200	2.0	800	800	350	10	15	150	70
60	1.2	1.4	15	2.0	200	2.0	800	800	350	10	15	150	70
50	1.1	1.3	15	1.4	150	2.0	1,200	1,200	280	15	12	150	45
60	1.1	1.3	15	1.5	180	2.0	1,200	1,200	300	15	12	150	50
60	1.1	1.3	15	1.6	180	2.0	1,200	1,200	280	15	12	150	55
60	1.1	1.3	15	1.6	180	2.0	800	800	280	15	12	150	55
60	1.0	1.2	13	1.6	180	2.0	800	800	280	10	12	150	55
70	1.5	1.6	17	2.2	400	2.2	1,200	1,200	320	30	15	175	65
95	1.6	1.8	20	2.1	280	2.6	1,200	1,200	355	15	19	200	75
90	1.6	1.7	20	2.1	260	2.6	1,200	1,200	340	15	16	200	75

[c] Retinol equivalents. 1 retinol equivalent = 1 μg retinol or 6 mg beta carotene.

[d] As cholecalciferol. 10 μg cholecalciferol = 400 IU of vitamin D.

[e] α-Tocopherol equivalents. 1 mg d-α tocopherol = 1 α-TE. See text for variation in allowances and calculation of vitamin E activity of the diet as α-tocopherol equivalents.

[f] 1 NE (niacin equivalent) is equal to 1 mg of niacin or 60 mg of dietary tryptophan.

Source: Reprinted with permission from *Recommended Dietary Allowances*. 10th Edition, © 1989 by the National Academy of Sciences. Published by National Academy Press, Washington, DC.

Appendix I. 1983 Metropolitan Height and Weight Tables

1983 Metropolitan height and weight tables are shown in Table I-1.

To make an approximation of frame size, extend the arm and bend the forearm upward at a 90-degree angle. Keep fingers straight and turn the inside of the wrist toward the body. If a caliper is available, use it to measure the space between the two prominent bones on either side of the elbow (medial and lateral humeral epicondyles). Without a caliper, place thumb and index finger on these two bones and measure the space between thumb and index finger against a ruler or tape mea-

Table I-1 Height and Weight Tables, Metropolitan 1983*

	Men				Women		
Height	Small Frame	Medium Frame	Large Frame	Height	Small Frame	Medium Frame	Large Frame
5'2"	128–134	131–141	138–150	4'10"	102–111	109–121	118–131
5'3"	130–136	133–143	140–153	4'11"	103–113	111–123	120–134
5'4"	132–138	135–145	142–156	5'0"	104–115	113–126	122–137
5'5"	134–140	137–148	144–160	5'1"	106–118	115–129	125–140
5'6"	136–142	139–151	146–164	5'2"	108–121	118–132	128–143
5'7"	138–145	142–154	149–168	5'3"	111–124	121–135	131–147
5'8"	140–148	145–157	152–172	5'4"	114–127	124–138	134–151
5'9"	142–151	148–160	155–176	5'5"	117–130	127–141	137–155
5'10"	144–154	151–163	158–180	5'6"	120–133	130–144	140–159
5'11"	146–157	154–166	161–184	5'7"	123–136	133–147	143–163
6'0"	149–160	157–170	164–188	5'8"	126–139	136–150	146–167
6'1"	152–164	160–174	168–192	5'9"	129–142	139–153	149–170
6'2"	155–168	164–178	172–197	5'10"	132–145	142–156	152–173
6'3"	158–172	167–182	176–202	5'11"	135–148	145–159	155–176
6'4"	162–176	171–187	181–207	6'0"	138–151	148–162	158–179

*Weight according to frame (ages 25 to 59) for men wearing indoor clothing weighing 5 lb, shoes with 1-inch heels; for women, indoor clothing weighing 3 lb, shoes with 1-inch heels.

Source: Reprinted with permission from the Metropolitan Life Insurance Company, New York.

Appendix I: 1983 Metropolitan Height and Weight Tables

sure. Compare this measurement with those in Table I-2, which lists elbow measurements for medium-framed men and women. Measurements lower than those listed indicate a small frame. Higher measurements indicate a large frame.

Table I-2 Height and Elbow Breadth for Men and Women

Height in 1-Inch Heels	Elbow Breadth
Men	
5'2"–5'3"	2½"–2⅞"
5'4"–5'7"	2⅝"–2⅞"
5'8"–5'11"	2¾"–3"
6'0"–6'3"	2¾"–3⅛"
6'4"	2⅞"–3¼"
Women	
4'10"–4'11"	2¼"–2½"
5'0"–5'3"	2¼"–2½"
5'4"–5'7"	2⅜"–2⅝"
5'8"–5'11"	2⅜"–2⅝"
6'0"	2½"–2¾"

Source: Reprinted with permission from Metropolitan Life Insurance Company, New York.

Index

A

Absorption, food allergy and, 37-38
Achlorhydria, osteoporosis and, 123
Acidophilus cultures, arthritis and, 8
Acidophilus therapy, colonic bacterial flora disorders and, 98-99
Acne
   iodine and, 307
   vitamin A and, 254
   zinc and, 332
Acrodermatitis enteropathica, zinc and, 332
Addison's disease, sodium/chloride and, 328
Additives, food
   cancer and, 19
   food intolerance and, 44-45
Aerobic exercise
   diabetes mellitus, 31
   weight loss/control and, 159-160
Aflatoxins
   cancer and, 17
   liver, 22
Airborne, carcinogens, 17
Alcohol
   abuse, *See* Alcoholics
   abusers, thiamine and, 265
   calcium and, 293
   calories and, 196
   cancer and, 19
      breast, 20
      colorectal, 21
      liver, 22
      lung, 22
   colorectal cancer and, 21
   drinking problems, signs of, 203
   gout and, 12
   hangover management, 204
   health benefits of, 203
   health hazards of, 202-203
   hypertension and, 76
   immunity and, 90
   lactation and, 135
   non-insulin-dependent diabetes and, 29
   nutrition and, 202-204
   osteoporosis and, 123
   pregnancy and, 134
   retinopathy and, 34
   tolerance, zinc and, 332
   vitamin B5 and, 272
Alcoholics
   folic acid and, 278
   magnesium and, 311
   molybdenum and, 317
   selenium and, 322
   thiamine and, 265
   vitamin A and, 254
   vitamin B12 and, 281
   vitamin C and, 285
Alfalfa tablets, vitamin K and, 264
Alimentary hypoglycemia, 83
Alkaline-ash foods, gout and, 12
Allergy
   challenge test, 40-41
   elimination,
      arthritis and, 10
      diets, 39-40
   food. *See* Food allergy
   prevention of, 41
   treatment of, 41
Almond oil, lipids and, 217
Aluminum
   antacids, manganese and, 313
   hydroxide, molybdenum and, 317
Alzheimer's disease, geriatric nutrition and, 60-61
Amenorrhea, athlete's nutrition and, 152
Amino acids, 239-247
   alcohol and, 203
   arginine/ornithine, 245-246
   athlete's nutrition and, 153
   branched-chain, 246-247
   immunity and, 87
   lysine, 239
   phenylalanine/tyrosine, 241-242

sulfur-containing, arthritis and, 10, 243-244
taurine, 244-245
tryptophan, 240-241
Amyotrophic lateral sclerosis, branched-chain amino-acids and, 246
Anaphylaxis
food allergy and, 35-36
sulfites and, 45
Anemia, 3-7
alcohol and, 202
athlete's nutrition and, 4, 152
clinical protocols, 3-7
etiologies/differential diagnosis of, 4
folic acid and, 278
incidence of, 3
laboratory workup, initial, 3-4
macrocytic normochromic, 6-7
clinical assessment of, 7
treatment of, 7
menorrhagia/metrorrhagia and, 64
microcytic hypochromic, 5-6
preconception nutrition and, 128
pregnancy and, 131
See also specific type of anemia
signs/symptoms of, 3
thiamine and, 265
vitamin B12 and, 280, 281
vitamin E and, 260
Angina pectoris, 24
magnesium and, 311
selenium and, 323
Anorexia, thiamine and, 265
Antacids
folic acid and, 278
geriatric nutrition and, 58
iron and, 308
molybdenum and, 317
osteoporosis and, 123
phosphate and, 55
vitamin B3 and, 271
Anthropometry, medical history/examination and, 173
Antiarthritic drugs, geriatric nutrition and, 57-58
Antibiotics, geriatric nutrition and, 59

Antibody tests, food allergy and, 38
Anticoagulant overdose, vitamin K and, 264
Anticonvulsants
folic acid and, 278
osteoporosis and, 123
Antihyperlipidemic medications, geriatric nutrition and, 58
Antihypertensives
folic acid and, 278
geriatric nutrition and, 58
vitamin B6 and, 274
Antioxidants
cancer and,
breast, 20
colorectal, 21
immunity and, 89
Anxiety
disorders, thiamine and, 265
premenstrual syndrome and, 141
Appetite
premenstrual syndrome and, 142
suppressants, weight loss/control and, 157
tryptophan and, 242
zinc and, 332
Arginine
athlete's nutrition and, 153
immunity and, 87
tissue healing and, 111
weight loss/control and, 159
Arginine/ornithine, 245-246
Arm muscle circumference, muscle mass determination and, 175
Arrhythmias, cardiac. *See* Cardiac arrhythmias
Arthritis, 8-12
clinical protocols, 8-11
nutritional therapies and, 8-10
rheumatoid. *See* Rheumatoid arthritis
selenium and, 323
tryptophan and, 242
vitamin B6 and, 276
zinc and, 332
Artificial fats, 222
Asbestos, cancer and, lung, 22
Aspartame, 208
food intolerance and, 43

Aspirin
  folic acid and, 278
  geriatric nutrition and, 57
  vitamin B3 and, 271
  vitamin C and, 285, 288
Asthma
  benzoic acid and, 44
  magnesium and, 312
  sulfites and, 45
  tartrazine and, 44
  vitamin C and, 286
Atherosclerosis, 13-14
  accelerating factors, 14
  atherogenic factors, 13-14
  clinical protocols, 13-14
  initiating factors, 13-14
  non-insulin-dependent diabetes, 30
  plaque regression, 14
  protective factors, 14
  selenium and, 325
  sodium/chloride and, 330
  vitamin C and, 285
Athletes
  chromium and, 297
  molybdenum and, 318
  potassium and, 320
  sodium/chloride and, 328
Athlete's nutrition
  body fat and, 146
  calories and, 145-146
  carbohydrate and, 147-148
  eating disorders and, 146
  ergogenic aids and, 153-154
  fats and, 149
  fluids/electrolytes and, 149
  minerals and, 152-153
  protein and, 148-149, 237
  vitamins and, 151
Athletic anemia, 4
Atrophic gastritis, folic acid and, 278
Autism, vitamin B6 and, 276
Autoimmune system, chronic disease of, microcytic hypochromic anemia and, 5
Autonomic dysfunction, alcohol and, 202
Avocado
  sulfites and, 45

B

Bacterial overgrowth syndrome, digestive impairments and, 57
Barbiturates, geriatric nutrition and, 58
Barley
  carbohydrates and, 208
  fiber and, 214
  indigestion and, 92
Beans
  carbohydrates and, 208
  fiber and, 212, 215
  indigestion and, 92
Bee pollen, athlete's nutrition and, 153
Behavior modification, weight loss/control and, 157-158
Benzene, cancer and, 18
Benzidine, cancer and, bladder, 20
Benzoic acid, 45
  food intolerance and, 44-45
Beriberi, thiamine and, 265
Beta carotene
  angina pectoris and, 24
  arthritis and, 10
  atherosclerosis and, 14
  cancer and,
    cervical, 20
    endometrial, 21
    lung, 22
  cervical dysplasia and, 62
  geriatric nutrition and, 52
  immunity and, 88
  vitamin A and, 253, 256
  vitamin E and, 254
Betaine hydrochloride, hypochlorhydria and, 94
Bile acids
  cancer and, 18
  carcinogen activation and, 15
Biliary disease, dietary fats and, 218
Biliary insufficiency, 96-97
Bioelectric impedance analysis, body fat determination and, 174
Bioflavonoids, 288-289
  cancer and, 20
  cataracts and, 34

dysmenorrhea and, 63
menopausal symptoms and, 65
menorrhagia/metrorrhagia and, 64
musculoskeletal trauma and, 110, 111
rheumatoid arthritis and, 11
Biotin, 282-283
Birth
defects, folic acid and, 278
low weight at, 134
Bisulfite preservatives, thiamine and, 265
Black currant oil, 229
premenstrual syndrome and, 144
Bladder, cancer, risk factors, 20
Bleeding, vitamin K and, 264
Bloating
premenstrual syndrome and, 141
sodium/chloride and, 327
Blood clotting
see also Thrombosis
vitamin C and, 286
vitamin E and, 261, 262
Blood pressure
calcium and, 294
copper and, 301
potassium and, 320
sodium/chloride and, 328
tryptophan and, 242
vitamin B3 and, 271
see also Hypertension
β-napthylamine, cancer and, bladder, 20
Body
composition analysis, calories and, 199
fat, determinations, medical history/ examination and, 174-175
mass index, calories and, 199
Bone(s)
alcohol and, 202
athlete's nutrition and, 152
densitometry, 176
loss,
calcium and, 294
molybdenum and, 318
vitamin K and, 264
marrow, disorders of, anemia and, 4
mass, calcium and, 293
selenium and, 325

Borage oil, 229
premenstrual syndrome and, 144
Boron, 290-291
osteoporosis and, 126
Bottle-feeding, folic acid and, 278
Bradycardia, potassium and, 320
Bran
calcium and, 292
copper and, 300
fiber and, 212
see also Fiber
irritable bowel syndrome and, 48
ulcerative colitis and, 49
zinc and, 331
Branched-chain amino-acids, 246-247
Breast cancer
alcohol and, 202
risk factors, 20
selenium and, 322, 323
simple sugars and, 207
vitamin D and, 258
vitamin E and, 260, 261
Breast congestion, premenstrual syndrome and, 141
Breast-feeding
allergies and, 139
fluoride and, 302
manganese and, 313
zinc and, 331
Brewer's yeast
chromium and, 296
diabetes mellitus, 31
folic acid and, 277
food intolerance and, 44
riboflavin and, 267
thiamine and, 264
vitamin B3 and, 269
vitamin B12 and, 280
Broad beans, gastrointestinal disease and, 43
Bronchial asthma, magnesium and, 312
Brown fat, obesity and, 120
Brown sugar, carbohydrates and, 205
Bruising
bioflavonoids and, 289
vitamin C and, 285
Burns, protein and, 237

C

Cabbage
  indigestion and, 92
  iodine and, 306
  juice, peptic ulcers and, 47
Cadmium
  cancer and, prostate, 23
  copper and, 300
  hypertension and, 79
  selenium and, 322
  zinc and, 331
Caffeine
  calcium and, 293
  cardiac arrhythmias and, 25
  hyperadrenalism and, 81
  hypertension and, 78
  lactation and, 135
  obesity and, 120
  osteoporosis and, 123
  potassium and, 319
  see also Coffee
Calcium, 291-295
  alcohol and, 203
  athlete's nutrition and, 152
  boron and, 290
  caffeine and, 293
  cancer and,
    colorectal, 21
    esophageal, 21
  dysmenorrhea and, 63
  fasting diets and, 156
  fracture healing and, 112
  geriatric nutrition and, 54
  high-protein/fat, low-carbohydrate dies, 156
  hypercholesterolemia and, 73
  lactation and, 135
  low-birth-weight and, 137
  manganese and, 313
  muscle cramps and, 108
  oxalate stones, 100
    management of, 100-101
  preconception nutrition and, 128
  pregnancy and, 130
  rheumatoid arthritis and, 11
  therapy,
    hypertension, 77-78
    osteoporosis, 127
Calories
  body,
    composition analysis and, 199
    mass index and, 199
  deficiency of, 200
  dense foods, 195
  dietary analysis and, 177
  empty, 196
  excess of, 200-201
  geriatric nutrition and, 50
  height tables and, 198-199
  metabolic rate and, 200
  nutrients value, 195
  pediatric growth charts and, 198
  requirements for,
    ages 19 to 50 years, 196
    diet-induced thermogenesis, 197
    estimating total requirements for, 198
    physical activity, 197
    resting metabolic rate, 196-197
  US adult intake of, 195
  weight tables and, 198-199
Cancer
  alcohol and, 202
  bladder, risk factors, 20
  breast,
    risk factors, 20
    simple sugars and, 207
  cervical, risk factors, 20
  clinical protocols, 15-23
  colon, fiber and, 213
  colorectal, risk factors, 21
  copper and, 300
  endometrial, risk factors, 21
  esophageal, risk factors, 21
  folic acid and, 278
  kidney, risk factors, 21
  liver, 22
  lungs, 22
  microcytic hypochromic anemia and, 5
  natural history of, 15-16
  obesity and, 200
  ovaries, 22

pancreas, 22
promoters of, 18-20
prostate, 23
protein and, 237
selenium and, 322, 323
skin, 23
stomach, 23
vitamin A and, 254
vitamin B12 and, 281
vitamin C and, 285, 286
vitamin E and, 260, 261
zinc and, 332
see also specific type of cancer
Candidiasis
systemic, 66-68
vaginal, 66
Canola oil, lipids and, 217
Capillary fragility, bioflavonoids and, 289
Carbohydrates, 205-211
athlete's nutrition and, 147-148
complex, 208-211
Crohn's disease and, 49
diabetes mellitus, 31
digestive impairments and, 57
geriatric nutrition and, 50-51
immunity and, 86
infant formulas and, 136
insulin-dependent diabetes and, 29
loading, 147
obesity and, 120
simple sugars and, 205-207
thiamine and, 265
ulcerative colitis and, 49
Carcinogens
airborne, 17
bioflavonoids and, 289
foodborne, 16-17
natural history of cancer and, 15-16
vitamin C and, 286
waterborne, 17
Carcinoid syndrome, vitamin B3 and, 269
Cardiac
arrhythmias, 24-25
alcohol and, 202
clinical protocols, 24-25
fiber and, 213

high-protein/fat, low-carbohydrate diets, 156
magnesium and, 311, 312
potassium and, 320
vitamin B3 and, 271
vitamin B5 and, 272
failure, thiamine and, 265
function, magnesium and, 312
medications, geriatric nutrition and, 58
Cardiomyopathy
alcohol and, 202
selenium and, 323
Cardiovascular
degeneration, copper and, 300
disease,
clinical protocols, 24-27
simple sugars and, 206
selenium and, 322
see also Heart
Carnitine
diabetes mellitus, 32
lipids and, 234-235
Carotenoids
see also Beta carotene
cancer and, 20
geriatric nutrition and, 52
Carpal tunnel syndrome, vitamin B6 and, 275
Cataracts
diabetes mellitus and, 34
riboflavin and, 267
vitamin C and, 285
vitamin E and, 261
Caucasoid race, endometrial cancer and, 21
Celiac sprue, 42
Cell-mediated and cellular immunity
iron and, 309
zinc and, 332
Cell-mediated reaction, food allergy and, 37
Central nervous system
alcohol and, 202
vitamin B3 and, 269
Cephalosporin, geriatric nutrition and, 59
Cerebral thrombosis, alcohol and, 203
Cervical
cancer,
risk factors, 20

vitamin C and, 285, 286
dysplasia, 62
  folic acid and, 279
Children, zinc and, 332
Chloride, 325-329
Chocolate
  breast-feeding and, 137
  food intolerance and, 44
  lysine and, 239
Cholecalciferol. *See* Vitamin D
Cholecystitis, 43
Cholesterol, 222-223
  breast-feeding and, 137
  cancer and, lung, 22
  chromium and, 297
  colorectal cancer and, 21
  copper and, 300
  dietary analysis and, 178
  fasting diets and, 156
  fiber and, 215
  low-birth-weight and, 137
  lysine and, 239
  microangiopathy and, 34
  retinopathy and, 34
  score, 224-227
  vitamin B3 and, 270
  vitamin B5 and, 272
  vitamin C and, 286
  zinc and, 333
Cholestyramine resin, geriatric nutrition and, 58
Choline
  fibrocystic breast disease and, 64
  lipids and, 230-232
  Parkinson's disease and, 61
Chondroitin sulfate, connective tissue repair
    and, 112
Chromate, cancer and, lung, 22
Chromium, 296-298
  geriatric nutrition and, 54
  hypoglycemia and, 84
  non-insulin-dependent diabetes and, 29
Chromosome breakage, folic acid and, 278
Cider, boron and, 290
Cirrhosis, liver, 202
  folic acid and, 278
  sodium/chloride and, 327

Citrate, athlete's nutrition and, 154
Clams
  cholesterol and, 222
  vitamin B12 and, 280
Claudication, intermittent, clinical protocols, 26
Cleft palate, folic acid and, 278
Clofibrate, geriatric nutrition and, 58
Clotting
  blood,
    vitamin C and, 286
    vitamin E and, 261, 262
Cobalamin, 280-282
  serum, macrocytic normochromic anemia
      and, 7
Cocaine, tryptophan and, 242
Cocoa
  bioflavonoids and, 288
  breast-feeding and, 137
Coconut oil, lipids and, 217
Cod liver oil
  vitamin D and, 257
  see also Fish oils
Coenzyme Q
  angina pectoris and, 24
  athlete's nutrition and, 153
  congestive heart failure and, 25
  diabetes mellitus, 32
  hypertension and, 79
Coffee
  bioflavonoids and, 288
  cancer and, ovarian, 22
  cholesterol and, 72
  iron and, 308
  magnesium and, 311
  thiamine and, 265
  see also Caffeine
Cognitive impairment, vitamin B12 and, 281
Colchicine, geriatric nutrition and, 58
Colds, vitamin C and, 285
Colestipol, geriatric nutrition and, 58
Colitis, ulcerative, 49
Collards, magnesium and, 310
  see also Vegetables
Colon
  arthritis and, 8
  bacteria in, protein and, 238

cancer,
    calcium and, 294
    fiber and, 213
    selenium and, 322
    polyps, vitamin C and, 286
Colonic bacterial flora disorders, 97-99
Colonic bacterial hyperproliferation, 97-99
Colorectal cancer
    risk factors, 21
    vitamin D and, 258
Complex carbohydrates, 208-211
Computerized diet analysis, 172
Conception, vitamin B6 and, 276
Congenital anomalies, 134
Congestive heart failure, 25
    clinical protocols, 25
    fasting diets and, 156
Connective tissue
    copper and, 300
    repair of, 112
    selenium and, 325
Constipation
    digestive impairments and, 57
    fiber and, 213
    high-protein/fat, low-carbohydrate diets, 156
Contraceptives
    cancer and,
        cervical, 20
        ovarian, 22
    folic acid and, 278
    gynecologic disorders and, 65
    osteoporosis and, 123
    preconception nutrition and, 128
    vitamin B6 and, 274, 275, 276
    vitamin C and, 285
Convulsive disorders, manganese and, 313
Copper, 299-301
    arthritis and, 10
    cancer and,
        breast, 20
        kidney, 21
        liver, 22
    geriatric nutrition and, 54

    low-birth-weight and, 137
    non-insulin-dependent diabetes, 32
    pregnancy and, 130
    tissue healing and, 111
    zinc and, 331, 333
Corn
    breast-feeding and, 137
    carbohydrates and, 205, 208
    fiber and, 215
    oil, lipids and, 217
    syrup, 205
Corneal vascularization, riboflavin and, 267
Coronary
    thrombosis,
        alcohol and, 203
        clinical protocols, 25-26
    vasospasm, magnesium and, 312
Corticosteroids
    geriatric nutrition and, 58
    osteoporosis and, 123
    potassium and, 319
Cortisone, vitamin D and, 257
Cottonseed oil, lipids and, 217
Cough, iodine and, 307
Cramps, foot, vitamin E and, 261
Cretinism, iodine and, 306
Crohn's disease, 48-49
Cruciferous vegetables, cancer and, 20
Cushing's disease
    osteoporosis and, 123
    potassium and, 319
Cyclamate, 208
Cysteine, 243
    alcohol and, 203
Cystic fibrosis, 42
    dietary fats and, 218
    pancreatic insufficiency and, 95
    vitamin A and, 254
    vitamin E and, 260
Cystine
    infant formulas and, 136
    stones, 101
Cytochromes, athlete's nutrition and, 153
Cytotoxic test, food allergy and, 38

D

Dairy products
  calcium and, 292
  food intolerance and, 43
  iodine and, 305
  osteoporosis and, 126
  protein and, 236, 237
  zinc and, 330
  see also specific dairy product
Dark leafy vegetables. *See* Vegetables
Degenerative joint disease, manganese and, 314
Dehydration
  athlete's nutrition and, 149
  fasting diets and, 156
Dental caries
  fluoride and, 302
  selenium and, 324
  simple sugars and, 206
Dental erosion, vitamin C and, 288
Deoxyribonucleic acid (DNA). *See* DNA
Depression
  folic acid and, 278
  hyperadrenalism and, 81
  premenstrual syndrome and, 142
  thiamine and, 265
  tryptophan and, 240
  vitamin B6 and, 275
Dermatitis
  biotin and, 283
  tryptophan and, 242
DES. *See* Diethylstilbesterol
Detoxification, vitamin B3 and, 270
Dextrose, 205
DHA. *See* Docosahexaenoic acid
Diabetes/diabetes mellitus
  alcohol and, 202
  calcium and, 293
  cancer and, endometrial, 21
  chromium and, 296, 297, 298
  complications, clinical protocols, 33-34
  cysteine and, 244
  diet, hypoglycemia and, 84
  folic acid and, 279
  gestational, 132-133
  hypoglycemia and, 83
  insulin-dependent, clinical protocols, 28
  magnesium and, 311
  manganese and, 313
  non-insulin-dependent, clinical protocols, 29-32
  obesity and, 200
  osteoporosis and, 123
  preconception nutrition and, 128
  vitamin A and, 254
  vitamin B6 and, 274, 276
  vitamin C and, 285
Diarrhea
  copper and, 299
  fiber and, 216
  magnesium and, 311, 312
  potassium and, 319
  sodium/chloride and, 328
  taurine and, 246
  vitamin B3 and, 271
  vitamin B5 and, 274
  vitamin C and, 287
Diet
  aids, 157-158
  allergy eliminating, 39-40
  analysis,
    calories and, 177
    computerized, 172
    deficiencies/excesses, 178-179
    exchange system and, 184
    micronutrients and, 179
    protein and, 179
  arthritis and, 8-10
  fiber. *See* Fiber
  history, 171-172
  hypoglycemia and, 84
  osteoarthritis and, 11-12
  pregnancy and, 129
  prescription, exchange system and, 184-185
  recall inventory, 171
  therapy. *See* Nutrition therapies

weight loss/control and, 155-156
Diethylstilbesterol (DES)
　cancer and, 18
　　cervical, 20
Dieting, osteoporosis and, 123
Digestion
　food allergy and, 37
　inhibitors, weight loss/control and, 158
Digitalis
　geriatric nutrition and, 58
　magnesium and, 311
Digoxin, geriatric nutrition and, 58
Dimethylglycine (DMG)
　athlete's nutrition and, 154
　immunity and, 90
Diuresis, potassium and, 319
Diuretics
　geriatric nutrition and, 58
　hypertension and, 79
　magnesium and, 311, 312
　osteoporosis and, 123
　potassium and, 319, 320
　therapy using, sodium/chloride and, 327
　thiamine and, 265
Diverticulitis, digestive impairments and, 57
Diverticulosis, fiber and, 213
Dizziness
　hyperadrenalism and, 81
　MSG and, 45
　selenium and, 324
DL-Phenylalanine
　osteoarthritis and, 12
　rheumatoid arthritis and, 12
　tryptophan and, 242
DMG. *See* Dimethylglycine
DNA, carcinogen binding to, 15
Docosahexaenoic acid (DHA),
　hypercholesterolemia and, 73
Drinking problems, signs of, 203
Drowsiness, hyperadrenalism and, 81
Drug detoxification, vitamin B3 and, 270
Drugs, lactation and, 135
Dysmenorrhea, 62-63

E

Eclampsia, 132
EDB, cancer and, 17
Edema
　protein and, 237
　thiamine and, 265
Eggplant, magnesium and, 310
Elderly
　calcium and, 292
　chromium and, 296
　copper and, 300
　iron and, 308
　potassium and, 321
　thiamine and, 265
　vitamin B6 and, 274, 275
　vitamin B12 and, 281
　vitamin D and, 257, 258
　vitamin K and, 263
　zinc and, 331
Electrolytes
　athlete's nutrition and, 149, 150
　digestive impairments and, 57
　muscle cramps and, 107
　sodium/chloride and, 329
ELISA, allergies and, 38
Emotional stress, cancer and, 19
Emphysema, copper and, 300
Empty calories, 196
Encephalopathy, thiamine and, 265
Endocrine system, chronic disease of,
　microcytic hypochromic anemia and, 5
Endometrial cancer, risk factors, 21
Endorphin, premenstrual syndrome and, 143
Endurance, molybdenum and, 318
Enteritis, regional. *See* Chron's disease
Environmental health history, 170-171
Environmental toxins, tryptophan and, 243
Enzyme-linked immunosorbent (ELISA),
　allergies and, 38
Enzymes
　liver, carcinogen activation and, 15
　pancreatic insufficiency and, 95

Eosinophilia-myalgia syndrome, tryptophan and, 241
Epilepsy
  manganese and, 313
  taurine and, 245
  vitamin E and, 260
Epileptic medications, vitamin D and, 257
Ergogenic aids, athlete's nutrition and, 153-154
Erythrocyte hemolysis test, vitamin E and, 261
Esophageal cancer
  riboflavin and, 267
  risk factors, 21
  vitamin C and, 285
Estrogen
  calcium and, 294
  cancer and,
    breast, 20
    cervical and, 20
    endometrial, 21
  gynecologic disorders and, 65
  osteoporosis and, 127
  premenstrual syndrome and, 142
  vitamin B6 and, 274
Ethylene dibromide (EDB), cancer and, 17
Evening primrose oil. *See* Primrose oil
Exercise
  calcium and, 292
  carbohydrate during, 148
  chromium and, 296
  hypertension and, 78
  magnesium and, 311
  obesity and, 121
  weight loss/control and, 159-160
  weight-bearing, osteoporosis and, 126, 127
Eyes
  riboflavin and, 267
  vitamin E and, 260

F

Family health history, 170
FAST, allergies and, 38
Fasting
  diets, 156
  hypoglycemia, 81-82
Fasting plasma glucose
  carbohydrates and, 209-210
  diabetes mellitus and, 30
Fat malabsorption syndrome, 218
  vitamin D and, 257
  vitamin E and, 260
Fatigue
  high-protein/fat, low-carbohydrate diets, 156
  iron and, 308
  migraine headache and, 103
  premenstrual syndrome and, 142
  tryptophan and, 241
  vitamin B5 and, 272
Fats
  arthritis and, 10
  athlete's nutrition and, 149
  breast-feeding and, 137
  calories and, 196
  cancer and,
    lung, 22
    ovarian, 22
  cholecystitis and, 43
  dietary,
    analysis and, 178
    cancer and, 18
  digestive impairments and, 57
  geriatric nutrition and, 50-51
  health and, 218-220
  hypercholesterolemia and, 71-72
  hypertension and, 77
  immunity and, 86-87, 87
  indigestion and, 92
  insulin-dependent diabetes and, 29
  low-birth-weight and, 137
  non-insulin-dependent diabetes, 31
  obesity and, 120
  occurrence of, 217-218
  percent of in oils, 219
  polyunsaturated, arthritis and, 10
  retinopathy and, 34

substitutes, weight loss/control and, 158
  unnatural, 221-222
Fava beans, gastrointestinal disease and, 43
Feingold diet, neurologic development and,
  139-140
Fermented foods, food intolerance and, 44
Ferritin, serum, iron-deficiency anemia and, 6
Ferulic acid (FRAC), athlete's nutrition and,
  153
Fetal
  abnormalities, alcohol and, 202
  mortality/morbidity, 133
Fiber, 212-216
  breast-feeding and, 137
  cancer and,
    breast, 20
    colorectal, 21
    endometrial, 21
  colonic bacterial flora disorders and, 98
  dietary analysis and, 178
  geriatric nutrition and, 50-51
  hypercholesterolemia and, 72
  insoluble, 213-214
  irritable bowel syndrome and, 48
  non-insulin-dependent diabetes, 31
  osteoporosis and, 123
  selenium and, 324
  soluble, 214-216
  supplements, weight loss/control and, 157
  total dietary, 212
  weight loss/control and, 158
Fibrocystic breast disease, 63-64
  cancer and, 20
  iodine and, 306
  vitamin E and, 261
Fish
  cancer and, esophageal, 21
  canned, food intolerance and, 44
  cholesterol and, 222
  molybdenum and, 317
  proteus and, 45
  selenium and, 321
  vitamin B6 and, 274
Fish oils
  angina pectoris and, 24
  coronary thrombosis and, 26
  hypercholesterolemia and, 73

hypertension and, 77
immunity and, 87
intermittent claudication and, 26
see also Omega-3 fatty acids
non-insulin-dependent diabetes, 32
prevention/treatment of, 106
vitamin A and, 254
vitamin D and, 257, 259
Flatulence, digestive impairments and, 57
Fluid intake, gout and, 12
Fluids, athlete's nutrition and, 149
Fluoride, 301-303
  selenium and, 324
Fluoroallergosorbent (FAST), allergies and,
  38
Fluoxetine hydrocholoride, tryptophan and,
  241
Flushing, vitamin B3 and, 271
Folate
  erythrocyte, macrocytic normochromic
    anemia and, 7
  serum, macrocytic normochromic anemia
    and, 7
Folic acid, 277-280
  alcohol and, 202, 203
  anemia and, 4
  cancer and, cervical, 20
  cervical dysplasia and, 62
  digestive impairments and, 57
  geriatric nutrition and, 52
  immunity and, 88
  macrocytic normochromic anemia and, 7
  preconception nutrition and, 128
  pregnancy and, 130
Food
  calorie dense, 195
  cancer and, liver, 22
  frequency assessment, 172
  high fat, 217-218
  migraine headache and, 103, 105
  sweeteners, 205-206
Food additives
  cancer and, 19
  food intolerance and, 44-45
Food allergy
  clinical protocols, 35-41
    challenge test, 40-41

diets for, 39-40
  immune reaction caused, 35-37
  laboratory tests for, 38-39
  predisposing conditions, 37-38
  prevention, 41
  treatment, 41
 questionnaire, 36
Food groups
 animal proteins, 180
 diary products, 171, 180
 exchange system, 183-191
  choices in, 186-189
  optimal health and, 190
  work sheet, 191
 fruit, 181
 nutrition density in, 182
 vegetables, 181
 whole-grain products, 181
Food intolerance
 clinical protocols, 42-45
  food additives causing, 44-45
  gastrointestinal disease, 42-43
  maldigestion disorders, 42
  metabolic defects, 43
  microorganism contamination causing, 45
  natural substances causing, 44
  psychologic reactions, 43
Foodborne carcinogens, 16-17
Foot, cramps, vitamin E and, 261
Formulas, infant
 carnitine and, 234
 fluoride and, 302
 infant nutrition and, 136
FRAC, athlete's nutrition and, 153
Fractures, healing of, 112
Free-radical pathology
 arthritis and, 10
 iron and, 310
 selenium and, 322, 323
 zinc and, 332
Fructose, 205
 copper and, 300
 diabetes mellitus, 31
 obesity and, 120
Fungicides, cancer and, 17
Furosemide, thiamine and, 265

G

Galactosemia, 43
 food intolerance and, 43
Gallbladder
 cancer and, colorectal, 21
 diseases, obesity and, 200
Gallstones
 alcohol and, 203
 fiber and, 216
 taurine and, 245
Gamma-radiation, cancer and, lung, 22
Garlic
 cancer and, 20
 coronary thrombosis and, 26
 hypercholesterolemia and, 73
Garlic breath order, selenium and, 324
Gas fumes, cancer and, lung, 22
Gastric
 cancer, vitamin C and, 285
 secretagogues, peptic ulcers and, 47
 ulcers,
  vitamin A and, 254
  zinc and, 332
Gastritis, alcohol and, 202
Gastrointestinal cancer, alcohol and, 202
Gastrointestinal diseases, 42-43
 clinical protocols, 46-49
  Crohn's disease, 48-49
  hiatal hernia, 46
  irritable bowel syndrome, 48-49
  peptic ulcer, 46-47
  reflux esophagitis, 46
  regional enteritis, 48-49
  ulcerative colitis, 49
 substances causing, 47
 zinc and, 331
Gastrointestinal distress
 copper and, 301
 iron and, 309
Gastrointestinal irritation
 folic acid and, 278
 selenium and, 324
 vitamin B3 and, 269
 vitamin B12 and, 281
Gastrointestinal remedies, geriatric nutrition and, 58

Gastrointestinal tract, maldigestion disorders and, 42
Genitals, riboflavin and, 267
Genitourinary tract, cancer of, selenium and, 322
Geriatric nutrition, 50-61
  calories and, 50
  carbohydrates and, 50-51
  dietary fiber and, 50-51
  drug-nutrient interactions and, 57-59
  fats and, 50-51
  health conditions affecting, 56-57
  mineral needs and, 54-56
  protein and, 51
  senile dementia and, 59-61
  vitamins and, 52-53, 53
  water and, 51
Germanium, 303-305
  immunity and, 90
Gestational diabetes, 132-133
  vitamin B6 and, 276
Ginseng therapy, menopausal symptoms and, 65
Glandulars, athlete's nutrition and, 153
Glossitis, folic acid and, 278
Glucomannan, non-insulin-dependent diabetes and, 31
Glucosamine, osteoarthritis and, 11
Glucose, 205
  6-phosphate dehydrogenase deficiency, food intolerance and, 43
  fasting diets and, 156
  fasting plasma, diabetes mellitus and, 30
  insulin tolerance test, 32, 210
  intolerance, fasting diets and, 156
  metabolism, premenstrual syndrome and, 143
  random plasma, diabetes mellitus and, 29
  tolerance,
    chromium and, 54, 297
    fiber and, 215
    gestational diabetes and, 132
    impaired, clinical protocols, 32-33
    sodium/chloride and, 330
    thiamine and, 265
    vitamin B3 and, 271
    zinc and, 332
    vitamin C and, 288
Glutamic acid hydrochloride, 94
Glutamine
  Crohn's disease and, 49
  immunity and, 87
  peptic ulcers and, 47
Glutathione, 243
Gluten foods, celiac sprue and, 42
Glycemic index foods, diabetes mellitus, 31
Glycine, tissue healing and, 111
Glycogen replacement, 147
Glycohemoglobin, 210-211
  diabetes mellitus and, 30
Glycosaminoglycan therapy, Crohn's disease and, 49
Glycosylated hemoglobin A, 210-211
Goiter, iodine and, 306
Gonyaulax catenella, food intolerance and, 45
Gout
  clinical protocols, 12
  high-protein/fat, low-carbohydrate diets, 156
  molybdenum and, 316
  nutritional therapies for, 12
  obesity and, 201
  vitamin C and, 287
Growth hormone stimulants, weight loss/control and, 159
Guar gum, non-insulin-dependent diabetes, 31
Gums
  disease of, simple sugars and, 206
  vitamin C and, 285
Gynecologic disorders, 62-68
  cervical dysplasia, 62
  dysmenorrhea, 62-63
  fibrocystic breast disease, 63-64
  obesity and, 200-201

H

Hair loss, biotin and, 283
Hangover management, 204
Hartnup's disease, vitamin B3 and, 269

Headache
  hyperadrenalism and, 81
  iodine and, 307
  MSG and, 45
  premenstrual syndrome and, 142
  tryptophan and, 242
  vitamin B3 and, 271
Heart
  attack, magnesium and, 311
  disease,
    alcohol and, 202
    magnesium and, 311
    obesity and, 200
    selenium and, 322
  failure, sodium/chloride and, 327, 328
  thiamine and, 265
Heavy metals
  hypertension and, 79
  selenium and, 323
Height tables, calories and, 198-199
Hemachromatosis, iron and, 310
Hemolytic anemia
  folic acid and, 278
  red blood cell loss and, 4
  vitamin E and, 260
Hemorrhage
  microcytic hypochromic anemia and, 5
  red blood cell loss and, 4
Hemorrhoids, fiber and, 213
Hepatitis B, cancer and, liver, 22
Herbicides, cancer and, 17
Herpes simplex, lysine and, 239
Herpes virus, taurine and, 246
Hiatal hernia, 46
  fiber and, 213
High complex-carbohydrate, low fat diet, 156
High-density lipoprotein deficiency, 74
High-fiber diet, weight loss/control and, 158
High-protein/fat, low-carbohydrate diet, 156
Histamine, food intolerance and, 44
Histamine blockers, geriatric nutrition and, 58
Histamine-releasing agents, food intolerance and, 44
Hives
  benzoic acid and, 44
  tartrazine and, 44
Homocystine, vitamin B6 and, 275
Homogenized milk, atherosclerosis and, 14
Honey, 206
  carbohydrates and, 205
Hormones, cancer and, 18
Horsetail herb, selenium and, 325
Hospitals, geriatric nutrition and, 57
Human chorionic gonadotropin, weight loss/control and, 159-160
Hydralazine, geriatric nutrition and, 58
Hydrochloric acid, maldigestion disorders and, 42
Hydrogenated fats, 221
Hydrostatic weighing, body fat determination and, 174
Hydroxyapatite, osteoporosis and, 127
Hyperadrenalism, hypoglycemia and, 81
Hypercholesterolemia, 69-74
  dietary fats and, 71-72
  dietary fiber and, 72
  evaluation of, 69-70
  incidence of, 69
  nutrient deficiencies and, 72
  therapeutic overview of, 70-71
  therapeutic supplements and, 73
Hyperlipidemia, obesity and, 200
Hypermetabolic disease, protein and, 237
Hyperparathyroidism, osteoporosis and, 123
Hypertension, 75-80
  alcohol and, 202
  drug/nutrient interactions, 79-80
  endometrial cancer and, 21
  evaluation, 75
  fiber and, 213
  magnesium and, 312
  nutrition therapies, 75-77
  obesity and, 200
  potassium and, 320
  preconception nutrition and, 128
  selenium and, 325
  sodium/chloride and, 327, 328
  taurine and, 244
  vitamin E and, 263

Hyperthyroidism
    osteoporosis and, 123
    vitamin D and, 258
Hypertriglyceridemia, 73
    alcohol and, 202
Hyperuricemia, high-protein/fat, low-carbohydrate diets, 156
Hypoallergenic
    food diet, 40
    formulas, 39
Hypocalcemia
    magnesium and, 311
    vitamin D and, 258
Hypochlorhydria, 94
    pernicious anemia and, 7
Hypoglycemia, 81-85
    alcohol and, 202
    chromium and, 297
    fasting, 81-82
    idiopathic, 83
    impaired glucose tolerance and, 32
    migraine headache and, 105
    reactive, 82-83
Hypokalemia, magnesium and, 311
Hyponatremia, 150
Hyporeflexia, magnesium and, 312
Hypotension
    fasting diets and, 156
    magnesium and, 312
Hypothalamic controls, obesity and, 117
Hypothalamus, obesity and, 118
Hypothyroidism
    iodine and, 306
    vitamin A and, 254

I

Ice cream, cholesterol and, 222
Immune
    complex formation, food allergy and, 37
    deficiency, alcohol and, 202
    function,
        vitamin A and, 254
        zinc and, 332
    response,
        food allergy and, 37
        vitamin B6 and, 275
        vitamin C and, 286
        vitamin E and, 53, 261
    system, selenium and, 323
Immunity
    adaptive, 85-86
    carbohydrates and, 86
    fats and, 86-87
    inborn, 85
    obesity and, 86
    suppression of, selenium and, 323
    very-low-calorie intake and, 86
    vitamin D and, 258
Impotence
    alcohol and, 202
    zinc and, 332
Indigestion
    biliary insufficiency, 96-97
    clinical assessment of, 91-92
    colonic bacterial flora disorders, 97-99
    differential diagnosis, 92-93
    foods causing, 92
    hypochlorhydria, 94
    incidence of, 91
    pancreatic insufficiency, 95-96
Infants
    fluoride and, 302
    premature, 134
        copper and, 299
    vitamin B6 and, 274
    vitamin C and, 284
    vitamin D and, 257
    vitamin E and, 260
    vitamin K and, 263
    see also Nutrition, infants
Infertility
    vitamin C and, 286
    zinc and, 332
Inflammation, iron and, 310
Inflammatory prostaglandins, bioflavonoids and, 289
Infrared interactance, body fat determination and, 175
Inosine, athlete's nutrition and, 154

Inositol
  diabetes mellitus and, 33
  lipids and, 232-233
Insect repellent, thiamine and, 265
Insoluble fiber, 213-214
Insomnia
  hyperadrenalism, 81
  tryptophan and, 240
Insulin
  chromium and, 297
  fasting levels, diabetes mellitus and, 30
Intermittent claudication
  clinical protocols, 26
  vitamin E and, 261
Intestinal bacterial synthesis, vitamin K and, 263
Intolerance, food. *See* Food intolerance
Invert sugar, 205
Iodine, 305-307
  deficiency, fibrocystic breast disease and, 64
  pregnancy and, 130
Ionizing radiation, cancer and, 17
Iron, 307-310
  absorption, vitamin C and, 285
  anemia and, 4
  arthritis and, 10
  athlete's nutrition and, 152
  carnitine and, 234
  geriatric nutrition and, 54-55
  immunity and, 89
  infant formulas and, 136
  lactation and, 135
  low-birth-weight and, 137
  manganese and, 313
  molybdenum and, 315
  pregnancy and, 129, 130
  zinc and, 331, 333
Iron-deficiency anemia, 6
  copper and, 300
  menorrhagia/metrorrhagia and, 64
  vitamin C and, 285
Irritability
  hyperadrenalism, 81
  premenstrual syndrome and, 141
Irritable bowel syndrome, 48
  fiber and, 213, 216

Irritants, cancer and, 19
Isoniazid
  geriatric nutrition and, 59
  vitamin B3 and, 269
Isotope dilution, body fat determination and, 175

J

Joint disease, manganese and, 314

K

Ketoacidosis, fasting diets and, 156
Ketones, fasting diets and, 156
Ketonuria, diabetes mellitus and, 29
Kidney disease
  branched-chain amino-acids and, 246
  calcium and, 293
  magnesium and, 311
  molybdenum and, 317
  osteoporosis and, 123
  sodium/chloride and, 328
  vitamin D and, 257
Kidney failure
  molybdenum and, 318
  potassium and, 321
Kidney stones, 100-101
  calcium and, 295
  cysteine and, 244
  magnesium and, 312
  vitamin B6 and, 275, 276
  vitamin C and, 287
Kidneys
  arthritis and, 9
  cancer of, risk factors, 21
  chronic disease of, microcytic hypochromic anemia and, 5
  magnesium and, 312
  protein and, 238

L

Lactase, maldigestion disorders and, 42
Lactation, 135
  folic acid and, 278

zinc and, 331
Lactobacillus acidophilus therapy
    colonic bacterial flora disorders and, 99
    irritable bowel syndrome and, 48
Lactose, 205
    intolerance, 207
Laryngeal cancer, vitamin C and, 285
Laxatives
    geriatric nutrition and, 58
    magnesium and, 311
L-Carnitine
    angina pectoris and, 24
    intermittent claudication and, 26
L-dopa
    bacteria in, 238
    geriatric nutrition and, 61
    vitamin B6 and, 52, 277
Lead
    hypertension and, 79
    toxicity, thiamine and, 265
Lecithin, hypercholesterolemia and, 73
Leg cramps, pregnancy and, 131
Lethargy, premenstrual syndrome and, 142
Leukotrienes, bioflavonoids and, 289
Levulose, 205
Linoleic acid, retinopathy and, 34
Lipid disorders, 69-74
Lipids/lipid factors, 217-235
    carnitine, 234-235
    cholesterol, 222-223
        score, 224-227
    choline, 230-232
    dietary fats and,
        health and, 218-220
        occurrence of, 217-218
        unnatural, 221-222
    inositol, 232-233
    omega-3 fatty acids, 227-229
    omega-6 fatty acids, 229-230
    plant sterols, 227
Lipotropics, arthritis and, 8
Liquid formula diets, 156
Lite salt, sodium/chloride and, 326
Liver
    alcohol and, 202
    arthritis and, 8
    biotin and, 282

cancer, 22
cholesterol and, 222
chronic disease of, microcytic
    hypochromic anemia and, 5
cirrhosis,
    alcohol and, 202
    sodium/chloride and, 327
    vitamin B3 and, 269
copper and, 299
disease,
    branched-chain amino-acids and, 246
    thiamine and, 265
    vitamin A and, 254
    vitamin E and, 260
enzymes, carcinogen activation and, 15
iron and, 307
protein and, 238
riboflavin and, 267
Lumbar disc prolapse, 110
Lungs
    arthritis and, 9
    cancer, 22
        selenium and, 322
    disease of, vitamin E and, 260
Lymphatic
    activity, arginine/ornithine and, 245
    cancer, selenium and, 322
Lysine, 239

M

Macrocytic normochromic anemia, 6-7
    clinical assessment of, 7
    treatment of, 7
Macular degeneration, zinc and, 332
Magnesium, 310-312
    alcohol and, 203
    boron and, 290
    cancer and, esophageal, 21
    cardiac arrhythmias and, 25
    congestive heart failure and, 25
    coronary thrombosis and, 26
    dysmenorrhea and, 63
    fasting diets and, 156
    fracture healing and, 112
    geriatric nutrition and, 55

Index

lactation and, 135
low-birth-weight and, 137
manganese and, 313
microangiopathy and, 34
molybdenum and, 317
muscle cramps and, 108
non-insulin-dependent diabetes, 32
preconception nutrition and, 128
premenstrual syndrome and, 144
selenium and, 324
therapy, hypertension, 78
Magnetic resonance, body fat determination and, 175
Malabsorption syndromes
  folic acid and, 278
  iron and, 308
  molybdenum and, 317
  osteoporosis and, 123
  preconception nutrition and, 128
  protein and, 237
  thiamine and, 265
  vitamin B12 and, 280
  vitamin K and, 263
Maldigestion
  disorders, 42
  secondary effects of, 93
Malignant melanoma, vitamin B6 and, 276
Manganese, 313-316
  arthritis and, 10
  connective tissue repair and, 112
  geriatric nutrition and, 55
  non-insulin-dependent diabetes, 32
  tissue healing and, 111
Manic-depressive illness, vitamin C and, 286
Mannitol, 208
Maple syrup, 206
  carbohydrates and, 205
Margarine
  liquid, lipids and, 217
  vitamin E and, 259
Marijuana, lactation and, 135
Mastalgia, premenstrual syndrome and, 141
Mean corpuscular volume (MCV), iron-deficiency anemia and, 6
Meats
  cancer and,
    breast, 20
    esophageal, 21
    pancreatic, 22
Medical history/examination
  health problems and, 169
  laboratory tests and, 176
  patient history and, 170-172
  physical tests and, 172-176
  preventive health care and, 169
Medications, geriatric nutrition and, 57-59
Megaloblastic anemia
  folic acid and, 278
  vitamin B12 and, 281
Melons, 92, 284, 310
Menaquinone. *See* Vitamin K
Menarche, cancer and, breast, 20
Menkes' kinky hair syndrome, copper and, 300
Menopause
  alcohol and, 202
  cancer and, 20
  symptoms, 65
Menorrhagia, 64-65
  vitamin A and, 254
Menstrual cramps, magnesium and, 311
Mental
  function, iron and, 308
  impairment, hyperadrenalism and, 81
  retardation,
    folic acid and, 279
    pregnancy and, 134
Mercury
  copper and, 300
  selenium and, 322
  zinc and, 331
Metabolic defects, 43
Metabolic rate
  calories and, 200
  fasting diets and, 156
  folic acid and, 278
  resting, 197
Metabolism, molybdenum and, 316
Metastasis, 16
Methionine, 243
  carnitine and, 234
  protein and, 237
Methyl xanthine, fibrocystic breast disease and, 64

Metrorrhagia, 64-65
Microangiopathy, diabetes mellitus and, 34
Microcirculatory disorders, bioflavonoids and, 289
Microcrystalline hydroxyapatite, fracture healing and, 112
Microcytic hypochromic anemia, 5-6
  treatment of, 6
Micronutrients
  dietary analysis and, 179
  supplements of, weight loss/control and, 157
  see also specific name of micronutrient
Midarm circumference, muscle mass determination and, 175
Migraine headache
  clinical assessment of, 103, 105
  etiology of, 102
  incidence of, 102
  prevention/treatment of, 105-106
  tryptophan and, 242
  work sheet, 104
Milk
  breast-feeding and, 137
  indigestion and, 92
  infant formulas and, 136
Millet, carbohydrates and, 208
Mineral oil, geriatric nutrition and, 58
Miscarriage, 130
Mixed-food conventional diet, weight control and, 155-156
Molasses, 205
  calcium and, 292
  carbohydrates and, 205
  iron and, 307
Molybdenum
  cancer and, esophageal, 21
  manganese and, 315
  selenium and, 324
Monoamine oxidase, tryptophan and, 242
Monosodium glutamate (MSG)
  food intolerance and, 45
  sodium/chloride and, 326
  vitamin B6 and, 275
Monounsaturated fats
  atherosclerosis and, 14
  cancer and, endometrial, 21

Mood swings, premenstrual syndrome and, 141
Morning sickness, 131
Motor dysfunction, vitamin B6 and, 277
Motor impairment, vitamin B12 and, 281
Mouth
  metallic taste in, selenium and, 324
  riboflavin and, 267
MSG
  food intolerance and, 45
  sodium/chloride and, 326
  vitamin B6 and, 275
Mucopolysaccharides, connective tissue repair and, 112
Mucosal irritants, peptic ulcers and, 47
Muscle
  cramps, 107-108
    calcium and, 294
    magnesium and, 311
  degeneration, selenium and, 323
  mass determinations, 175
  spasm, musculoskeletal trauma and, 112-113
  vitamin E and, 260
  wasting, protein and, 237
  weakness,
    magnesium and, 311
    potassium and, 320
    thiamine and, 265
Musculoskeletal trauma, 109-113
  inflammatory phase of, 109
  muscle spasm and, 112-113
  proliferative phase of, 111-112
Mutation, folic acid and, 278
Myocardial atrophy, fasting diets and, 156
Myocardial infarction
  clinical protocols, 27
  selenium and, 322
  thiamine and, 265

N

Narcolepsy, tryptophan and, 242
Nausea
  high-protein/fat, low-carbohydrate diets, 156

iodine and, 307
manganese and, 315
potassium and, 321
taurine and, 246
vitamin B3 and, 271
vitamin B6 and, 276
zinc and, 333
Neonatal abnormalities, alcohol and, 202
Nephropathy
diabetes mellitus and, 34
non-insulin-dependent diabetes, 30
Nerves
dysfunction of, vitamin B6 and, 275
vitamin B6 and, 275
vitamin E and, 260
Nervous tension, premenstrual syndrome and, 141
Nervousness, hyperadrenalism, 81
Neuritis, alcohol and, 202
Neuroglycopenia, hypoglycemia and, 81
Neurologic, impairment, hyperadrenalism and, 81
Neurologic disorders
vitamin B6 and, 277
vitamin B12 and, 281
vitamin E and, 260
Neuropathy
diabetes mellitus and, 33
non-insulin-dependent diabetes, 30
Neuroses, thiamine and, 265
Neutron activation, body fat determination and, 175
Neutropenia, copper and, 300
Neutrophils, hypersegmented, macrocytic normochromic anemia and, 7
Niacin, 269-271
cancer and, esophageal, 21
carnitine and, 234
diabetes mellitus, 32
dysmenorrhea and, 63
hypercholesterolemia and, 73
Niacinamide, 269-271
diabetes mellitus, 31
osteoarthritis and, 11
Nickel, cancer and, lung, 22
Nicotine, lactation and, 135
Nicotinic acid, peptic ulcers and, 47

Nightshade plants, arthritis and, 9
Nitrates
breast-feeding and, 137
cancer and,
bladder, 20
esophageal, 21
carcinogen activation and, 15
thiamine and, 265
Nitrites, cancer and, esophageal, 21
Nitrosamines
cancer and, 17
liver, 22
Nonsteroidal anti-inflammatory drugs, geriatric nutrition and, 57
Normocytic normochromic anemias, 4
Nucleotides, immunity and, 87
Numbness, vitamin B6 and, 277
Nutrition
alcohol and, 202-203, 203-204
athlete's, 145-54, *see also* Athlete's nutrition
considerations,
Alzheimer's dementia and, 60-61
Parkinson's disease and, 61
infants,
allergy prevention, 139
anemia monitoring, 139
breast feeding, 136
dental caries and, 140
formulas, 136
monitoring weight gain, 138
neurologic development, 139-140
normal growth, 138
optimal, 137
post-weaned, 137
preventing imbalances, 138
special situations, 138
lactation and, 135
preconception, 128
pregnancy and, 129-135
Nutritional insufficiencies, cancer and, 19-20

O

Oat bran
fiber and, 215
non-insulin-dependent diabetes, 31

Obesity
  appetite regulation and, 117-119
  body fat percentage and, 114-115
  breast cancer and, 20
  cancer and,
    colorectal, 21
    endometrial, 21
    kidney, 21
    prostate, 23
  defined, 200
  development influences on, 117
  environmental/psychologic factors, 119
  genetic influences on, 116
  gestational diabetes and, 132
  health risks of, 115-116
  immunity and, 86
  incidence of, 115
  intrinsic food factors, 119
  morbidity and, 116
  mortality and, 115
  non-insulin-dependent diabetes, 29, 30
  preconception nutrition and, 128
  thermogenic regulation, 119-121
  unusual causes of, 115
  weight for height and, 114
Occult blood, vitamin C and, 288
Octacosanol, athlete's nutrition and, 154
Odors, migraine headache and, 103
Olive oil
  LDL and, 72
  lipids and, 217
Omega-3 fatty acids
  cancer and,
    breast, 20
    colorectal, 21
    endometrial, 21
    pancreatic, 22
    prostate, 23
  infant formulas and, 136
  lipids and, 227-229
  rheumatoid arthritis and, 11
Omega-6 fatty acids
  cancer and,
    breast, 20
    colorectal, 21
    endometrial, 21
    pancreatic, 22
    prostate, 23
  endometrial cancer and, 21
  immunity and, 86
  lipids and, 229-230
  rheumatoid arthritis and, 11
Oral contraceptives
  breast cancer and, 20
  folic acid and, 278
  menopausal symptoms and, 65
  osteoporosis and, 123
  preconception nutrition and, 128
  vitamin B6 and, 274, 275, 276
  vitamin C and, 285
Oral glucose tolerance test, 210
  non-insulin-dependent diabetes, 30
Organ meats
  gout and, 12
Ornithine
  athlete's nutrition and, 153
  weight loss/control and, 159
Osteoarthritis
  clinical protocols, 11-12
  niacinamide and, 270
  nutritional therapies and, 11-12
  obesity and, 201
  selenium and, 325
Osteomalacia
  molybdenum and, 318
  vitamin D and, 258
Osteoporosis
  boron and, 290, 291
  calcium and, 293
  clinical assessment of, 122-126
    bone density studies, 126
    laboratory tests, 123
    risk factors, 122-123
  described, 122
  fluoride and, 302
  incidence/demographics of, 122
  manganese and, 313
  prevention, 126
  risk factor questionnaire, 124-125
  treatment, 126-127
  vitamin D and, 257
  vitamin K and, 53, 264

Ovaries
  cancer, 22
    selenium and, 322
Overweight, defined, 200
Oxalate, calcium and, 292
Oxalic acid, vitamin B6 and, 275
Oxidative tissue damage
  copper and, 300, 301
  zinc and, 332
Oxidized fats, 221-222
Ozone, selenium and, 322

P

Pain
  chronic, tryptophan and, 242
  sensitivity, tryptophan and, 240
Palm oil, lipids and, 217
Palpitations, premenstrual syndrome and, 142
Pancreatectomy, pancreatic insufficiency and, 95
Pancreatic
  cancer, 22
    selenium and, 322
  disease, dietary fats and, 218
  insufficiency, 95-96
    manganese and, 313
    pernicious anemia and, 7
Pancreatitis
  alcohol and, 202
  pancreatic insufficiency and, 95
Pangamic acid, athlete's nutrition and, 154
Pantothenic acid, 272-277
  tissue healing and, 111
Parkinsonian symptoms, manganese and, 315
Parkinson's disease
  bacteria in, 238
  geriatric nutrition and, 61
  vitamin B6 and, 52, 277
  vitamin E and, 261
Patient history, medical history/examination and, 170-172
Peanut oil, lipids and, 217
Peanuts, lysine therapy and, 239

Pectin, ulcerative colitis and, 49
Pediatric growth charts, calories and, 198
Pediatric neurologic/behavioral problems, 134-135
Pellagra, vitamin B3 and, 269
Penicillamine, geriatric nutrition and, 58
Peppermint oil, irritable bowel syndrome and, 48
Peptic ulcers, 46-47
  vitamin B3 and, 271
Periodontal disease
  folic acid and, 279
  osteoporosis and, 123
Peripheral
  neuritis, alcohol and, 202
  neuropathy, vitamin B6 and, 275
  paresthesias, thiamine and, 265
Pernicious anemia
  cobalamin and, 7
  vitamin B12 and, 280, 281
Personal health history, 170
Personality
  cancer and, 19
  disorders, tryptophan and, 240
Perspiration, sodium/chloride and, 328
Pesticides, cancer and, 17
Petechial hemorrhages, vitamin C and, 285
Phenobarbital, cancer and, liver, 22
Phenylalanine/tyrosine, 241-242
Phenylethylamine, food intolerance and, 44
Phenylketonuria
  food intolerance and, 43
  tryptophan and, 242
Phenytoin, geriatric nutrition and, 58
Phosphate
  geriatric nutrition and, 55
  molybdenum and, 318
Phosphoric acid, molybdenum and, 317
Phosphorus, 316-318
  boron and, 290
  fracture healing and, 112
  manganese and, 313
  microangiopathy and, 34
  molybdenum, 317
  molybdenum and, 318
  osteoporosis and, 123

preconception nutrition and, 128
zinc and, 331
Phylloquinone. *See* Vitamin K
Physical activity
   caloric requirements and, 197
   non-insulin-dependent diabetes, 31
Physical tests, medical history/examination and, 172-176
Phytate
   calcium and, 292
   manganese and, 313
Pica, pregnancy and, 131-132
Pickled foods
   cancer and, liver, 22
   sodium/chloride and, 326
Plant oils, lipids and, 217
Plant sterols, 227
Polyphosphate, molybdenum and, 317
Polyunsaturated fats
   arthritis and, 10
   obesity and, 120
Polyuria, sodium/chloride and, 328
Ponderosity index, body fat determination and, 175
Postepisiotomy pain, 110
Postmenopausal women
   boron and, 291
   calcium and, 292, 294
   vitamin K and, 263
Postprandial plasma glucose, 210
Postural hypotension, vitamin B5 and, 272
Potassium, 318-321
   cardiac arrhythmias and, 25
   congestive heart failure and, 25
   fasting diets and, 156
   geriatric nutrition and, 55-56
   muscle cramps and, 107
   non-insulin-dependent diabetes, 32
   therapy, hypertension, 77
Precompetition meals, 147-148
Preeclampsia, 132
Pregnancy
   anemia during, 131
   chromium and, 296
   complications during, 130-132
      avoiding, 133-135
   dietary needs during, 129-130
   folic acid and, 278, 279
   magnesium and, 311
   osteoporosis and, 123
   sodium/chloride and, 329
   supplements during, 130
   vitamin B6 and, 274, 275
   vitamin D and, 257
   weight gain goals, 129
   zinc and, 331
Premenopausal women
   calcium and, 294
   vitamin K and, 263
Premenstrual syndrome, 141-145
   magnesium and, 312
   vitamin B6 and, 275
   vitamin E and, 261
Preventive health care, medical history/examination and, 169
Primidone, geriatric nutrition and, 58
Primrose oil
   diabetes mellitus and, 33
   fibrocystic breast disease and, 64
   intermittent claudication and, 26
   premenstrual syndrome and, 144
Pritikin diet, 156
   hypertension and, 77
Prolactin, premenstrual syndrome and, 143
Proline, tissue healing and, 111
Prostaglandin
   dysmenorrhea and, 63
   inflammatory, bioflavonoids and, 289
   modification,
      arthritis and, 10
      rheumatoid arthritis and, 11
   premenstrual syndrome and, 143
Prostate
   cancer, 23
      selenium and, 322
   zinc and, 332
Protein, 236-238
   athlete's nutrition and, 148-149
   cancer and,
      breast, 20
      colorectal, 21
      esophageal, 21
      liver, 22
   colonic bacterial flora disorders and, 98

dietary,
    analysis and, 179
    cancer and, 19
  digestive impairments and, 57
  food,
    guide and, 180
    intolerance and, 43
  geriatric nutrition and, 51
  immunity and, 87
  indigestion and, 92
  infant formulas and, 136
  inflammatory, proteolytic enzymes and, 109
  insulin-dependent diabetes and, 29
  losing pathologies, 238
  non-insulin-dependent diabetes, 31
  obesity and, 120
  osteoporosis and, 123
  predigested,
    hypochlorhydria and, 94
    pancreatic insufficiency and, 95
  pregnancy and, 129
  vitamin E and, 259
Proteolytic enzymes, musculoskeletal trauma and, 109-110
Proteus, food intolerance and, 45
Prozac, tryptophan and, 241
Prunes, iron and, 307
Psoriasis
  folic acid and, 278
  vitamin A and, 254
  vitamin D and, 258
Psoriatic arthritis, zinc and, 332
Psychiatric
  disorders, vitamin B12 and, 281
  patients, vitamin C and, 285
Psychoactive medications, geriatric nutrition and, 58
Psyllium
  fiber and, 214
  irritable bowel syndrome and, 48
  non-insulin-dependent diabetes, 31
  ulcerative colitis and, 49
Purine
  gout and, 12
  metabolism, molybdenum and, 316
Pustular acne, zinc and, 332
Pyridoxine, 274-277

R

Radiation
  ionizing, cancer and, 17
  lung cancer and, 22
Radioallergosorbent, (RAST) test, 38
Raisins, vitamin B6 and, 274
Random plasma glucose, diabetes mellitus and, 29
Rapeseed oil, lipids and, 217
Rash
  benzoic acid and, 45
  iodine and, 307
  tartrazine and, 44
Reactive hypoglycemia, 82-83
Reflux esophagitis, 46
Regional enteritis, 48-49
Renal disease, chronic, protein and, 238
Respiratory depression, magnesium and, 312
Resting metabolic rate, 197
Retinol. *See* Vitamin A
Retinopathy
  diabetes mellitus and, 34
  non-insulin-dependent diabetes, 30
Retrolental fibroplasia, vitamin E and, 261
Rheumatic heart disease, vitamin E and, 263
Rheumatism, vitamin B6 and, 276
Rheumatoid arthritis
  clinical protocols, 11
  copper and, 300
  nutritional therapies for, 11
  osteoporosis and, 123
  prostaglandin modification and, 10
  tryptophan and, 242
  vitamin B5 and, 272, 273
  zinc and, 332
Riboflavin, 257-258
  cancer and, esophageal, 21
Rickets, vitamin D and, 258
Rifampin, geriatric nutrition and, 59
Rose hips, bioflavonoids and, 288
Royal jelly, athlete's nutrition and, 153

S

Saccharin, 208
  cancer and, 17
    bladder, 20

Safflower oil, lipids and, 217
Safrol, cancer and, liver, 22
Salt
  breast-feeding and, 137
  calcium and, 293
  dietary analysis and, 178-179
  esophageal cancer and, 21
  iodine and, 305
  osteoporosis and, 123
Saturated fats
  cancer and,
    breast, 20
    colorectal, 21
    pancreatic, 22
    prostate, 23
  obesity and, 120
Scurvy, vitamin C and, 287
Seaweed, iodine and, 305
Seborrheic dermatitis
  biotin and, 283
  riboflavin and, 267
Secretagogues, peptic ulcers and, 47
Seizures, MSG and, 45
Selenium, 321-324
  alcohol and, 203
  arthritis and, 10
  atherosclerosis and, 14
  cancer and, 20
  cervical dysplasia and, 62
  coronary thrombosis and, 26
  geriatric nutrition and, 55-56
  immunity and, 89
  tissue healing and, 111
Senile
  cataracts, riboflavin and, 267
  dementia, geriatric nutrition and, 59-61
Sensory impairment, vitamin B12 and, 281
Serum
  ferritin, iron-deficiency anemia and, 6
  fructosamine, 211
    diabetes mellitus and, 30
  tocopherol, 261
Sesame oil, lipids and, 217
Sexual activity, cervical cancer and, 20
Shave grass, silicon and, 325

Shellfish
  cholesterol and, 222
  food intolerance and, 44
  gonyaulax catenella and, 45
Shrimp
  cholesterol and, 222
Sickle-cell anemia, folic acid and, 278
Sideroblastic anemia, 6
Silicon, 324-325
Skeletal deformities, alcohol and, 202
Skin
  arthritis and, 9
  cancer, 23
    selenium and, 322
  germanium and, 305
  sun-damaged, vitamin A and, 254
  vitamin B3 and, 269
  vitamin E and, 260, 261
Skinfold calipers, body fat determination and, 174
Smell, zinc and, 332
Smog
  cancer and, lung, 22
  selenium and, 322
Smoking
  cancer and, 17
    bladder, 20
    cervical, 20
    kidney, 21
    pancreatic, 22
  esophageal cancer and, 21
  folic acid and, 278
  osteoporosis and, 123
  vitamin A and, 254
  vitamin B12 and, 281
  vitamin C and, 286
Sodium, 325-329
  bicarbonate, athlete's nutrition and, 154
  hypertension and, 76-77
  low-birth-weight and, 137
  non-insulin-dependent diabetes, 31
Solanaceae plants, arthritis and, 9
Sorbitol, 208
Soy
  oil, lipids and, 217

Soybeans, LDL and, 72
Spironolactone, hypertension and, 79
Spirulina, athlete's nutrition and, 153
Spontaneous abortion, 130
　folic acid and, 278
Sports
　drinks, 148, 150
　nutrition, 145-54, *see also* Athlete's
　　nutrition
Starch blockers, weight loss/control and, 158
Sterility, zinc and, 332
Sterols, plant, 227
Stomach
　bubble, weight loss/control and, 158
　cancer, 23
Stool, hemorrhage into, microcytic
　hypochromic anemia and, 5
Stress
　emotional, cancer and, 19
　hypertension and, 78-79
　migraine headache and, 103
　obesity and, 121
　osteoporosis and, 123
　tests, non-insulin-dependent diabetes and,
　　31
　tryptophan and, 242
　vitamin C and, 285
Stroke
　alcohol and, 202
　geriatric nutrition and, 59-60
　potassium and, 320
　selenium and, 322
Sublingual tests, food allergy and, 39
Substance abuse
　preconception nutrition and, 128
　pregnancy and, 134
Succinate, athlete's nutrition and, 153
Sucrose, 205
　obesity and, 120
Sudden death, fasting diets and, 156
Sugar
　breast-feeding and, 137
　calories and, 196
　carbohydrates and, 205
　chromium and, 296
　coronary thrombosis and, 26
　Crohn's disease, 49
　dietary analysis and, 178
　fluoride and, 302
　immunity and, 86
　intolerance, 206
　non-insulin-dependent diabetes, 31
　simple, 205-207
　　health risks of, 206-207
　substitutes, 207-208
　ulcerative colitis and, 49
　see also Sweets
Sulfasalazine, geriatric nutrition and, 58
Sulfate, molybdenum and, 315
Sulfites
　food intolerance and, 45
　molybdenum and, 315
　vitamin B12 and, 281
Sulfur-containing amino-acids, 243-244
Sunflower
　oil,
　　lipids and, 217
Support groups, weight loss/control and, 157
Surgery
　arginine/ornithine and, 245
　obesity and, 201
　substitutes, 159
　weight loss/control and, 158
Surgical wounds, zinc and, 332
Sweating, hyperadrenalism, 81
Sweets
　hyperadrenalism and, 81
　premenstrual syndrome and, 142
　see also Sugar
Sympathetic blocking agents, hypertension
　and, 80
Syncope, high-protein/fat, low-carbohydrate
　diets, 156
Systemic candidiasis, 66-68

T

Tachycardia, hyperadrenalism, 81
Tartrazine, food intolerance and, 44
Taste, zinc and, 332

Taurine, 244-245
  congestive heart failure and, 25
  hypertension and, 79
  infant formulas and, 136
  therapy, cardiac arrhythmias and, 25
Testosterone, alcohol and, 202
Tetracycline
  geriatric nutrition and, 59
  iron and, 310
  osteoporosis and, 123
Thalassemia minor, microcytic hypochromic anemia and, 5
Thermogenesis, diet-induced, 197
Thiamine
  alcohol and, 202
  see also Vitamin B
Thiazide, hypertension and, 79
Thrombophlebitis, vitamin E and, 261
Thrombosis
  coronary, clinical protocols, 25-26
  vitamin B5 and, 272
Thrombus, vitamin C and, 286
Thyroid
  calories and, 200
  disease, calcium and, 293
  hormones, weight loss/control and, 159
  iodine and, 307
  osteoporosis and, 123
Tobacco
  cancer and, 17, 20
  pancreatic, 22
Tocopherol. *See* Vitamin E
Tofu
  calcium and, 291, 292
  osteoporosis and, 126
Total-body electrical conductivity, body fat determination and, 175
Toxemia, 132
Toxic bowel syndrome, 97-99
Trace elements, immunity and, 90
Transferrin saturation, iron-deficiency anemia and, 6
Trauma
  arginine/ornithine and, 245
  branched-chain amino-acids and, 246
  manganese and, 314
  protein and, 238

Trembling, hyperadrenalism, 81
Tremors, magnesium and, 311
Triamterene, geriatric nutrition and, 58
Triceps skinfold measurements, muscle mass determination and, 175
Trichloromethanes, cancer and, bladder, 20
Triglycerides
  vitamin B3 and, 270
  vitamin B5 and, 272
Tryptophan, 240-241
  Parkinson's disease and, 61
Tumorigenesis, 16
Tumors
  arginine/ornithine and, 245
  protein and, 238
  vitamin D and, 258
Tyramine, food intolerance and, 44
Tyrosine
  athlete's nutrition and, 154
  infant formulas and, 136

U

Ulcerative colitis, 49
  colorectal cancer and, 21
Ulcers
  gastric, vitamin A and, 254
  peptic, 46-47
  zinc and, 332
Ultrasound measurement, body fat determination and, 174
Underwater weighing, body fat determination and, 174
Upper respiratory infections, zinc and, 332
Uric acid
  fasting diets and, 156
  stones, 101
  vitamin B3 and, 271
Urinary glucose, carbohydrates and, 209
Urine, hemorrhage into, microcytic hypochromic anemia and, 5

V

Vagina
  candidiasis of, 66
  yeast infections of, 66-68

Vanadium, 329-330
Varicose veins, fiber and, 213
Vasospastic angina, magnesium and, 311
Vasospastic circulation disorders, vitamin B3 and, 270
Vegan diet, diabetes mellitus and, 33
Vegetarians
   carnitine and, 234
   iron and, 308
   protein and, 237
   vitamin B12 and, 281
   vitamin D and, 257
   zinc and, 331
Very-low-calorie diet, 156
Vigor, loss of, tryptophan and, 241
Vinyl chloride, cancer and, liver, 22
Viruses, cancer and, 18
Visual disturbances, hyperadrenalism and, 81
Vitamin A, 253-256
   alcohol and, 202
   cancer and, 19
      bladder, 20
      cervical, 20
      esophageal, 21
      lung, 22
   cervical dysplasia and, 62
   geriatric nutrition and, 52
   immunity and, 88
   lactation and, 135
   menorrhagia/metrorrhagia and, 64
   migraine headache and, 103
   pancreatic insufficiency and, 95
   pregnancy and, 129, 130
   tissue healing and, 111
Vitamin B, 264-283
   alcohol and, 202, 203
   anemia and, 4
   biotin, 282-283
   cancer and, 19
   carnitine and, 234
   cobalamin, 280-282
   coronary thrombosis and, 26
   diabetes and, 33
   digestive impairments and, 57
   dysmenorrhea and, 63
   folic acid, 277-280
   geriatric nutrition and, 52
   immunity and, 88
   lactation and, 135
   niacin, 269-271
   niacinamide, 269-271
   non-insulin-dependent diabetes, 32
   pantothenic acid, 272-274
   Parkinson's disease and, 61
   preconception nutrition and, 128
   pregnancy and, 130
   premenstrual syndrome and, 144
   pyridoxine, 274-277
   retinopathy and, 34
   riboflavin, 267-268
   tissue healing and, 111
   tryptophan and, 242, 243
   see also B vitamins
Vitamin C, 284-288
   alcohol and, 202
   arthritis and, 10
   atherosclerosis and, 14
   cancer and, 17, 19
      cervical, 20
      esophageal, 21
   cervical dysplasia and, 62
   copper and, 300
   coronary thrombosis and, 26
   cysteine and, 244
   dysmenorrhea and, 63
   geriatric nutrition and, 53
   gout and, 12
   hypercholesterolemia and, 72
   hypertension and, 79
   immunity and, 88
   intermittent claudication and, 26
   lactation and, 135
   low-birth-weight and, 137
   menorrhagia/metrorrhagia and, 64
   microangiopathy and, 34
   musculoskeletal trauma and, 111
   non-insulin-dependent diabetes, 32
   pregnancy and, 129, 130
   protein and, 238
   retina and, 34
   selenium and, 323
   tissue healing and, 111
Vitamin D, 256-259
   alcohol and, 203

breast-feeding and, 136
calcium and, 292, 293
fracture healing and, 112
geriatric nutrition and, 53
immunity and, 88-89
low-birth-weight and, 137
osteoporosis and, 126, 127
pregnancy and, 130
Vitamin E, 259-263
angina pectoris and, 24
arthritis and, 10
atherosclerosis and, 14
athlete's nutrition and, 151
beta carotene and, 254
cancer and, 17, 19
cervical dysplasia and, 62
coronary thrombosis and, 26
dysmenorrhea and, 63
fibrocystic breast disease and, 64
geriatric nutrition and, 53
immunity and, 89
infant formulas and, 136
intermittent claudication and, 26
iron and, 309
low-birth-weight and, 137
menopausal symptoms and, 65
microangiopathy and, 34
osteoarthritis and, 11
premenstrual syndrome and, 144
rheumatoid arthritis and, 11
selenium and, 323
tissue healing and, 111
Vitamin K, 263-264
alcohol and, 202
geriatric nutrition and, 53
low-birth-weight and, 137
osteoporosis and, 126
Vomiting
potassium and, 319, 321
vitamin B3 and, 271
vitamin B6 and, 276
zinc and, 333

W

Waist/hip ratio, body fat determination and, 175
Water
copper and, 299
geriatric nutrition and, 51
iodine and, 305
kidney stones and, 100
molybdenum and, 315
muscle cramps and, 107
thiamine and, 265
vitamin C and, 285
Water fast, food allergy and, 39
Water intoxication, 150
Waterborne, carcinogens, 17
Weakness, hyperadrenalism, 81
Weight
preconception nutrition and, 128
tables, calories and, 198-199
Weight loss/control
calorie catabolism and, 159
calorie estimate and, 155
diet aids and, 157-158
diets for, 155-156
hypertension and, 75-76
non-insulin-dependent diabetes, 31
Wilson's disease, copper and, 301
Wine
sulfites and, 45
Withdrawal, premenstrual syndrome and, 142
Wound healing, 111
vitamin A and, 254
vitamin C and, 286
zinc and, 332

X

Xanthan gum, non-insulin-dependent diabetes, 31

Y

Yeast
  infections, vaginal, 66-68
  riboflavin and, 267
  zinc and, 330

Z

Zinc, 330-333
  alcohol and, 203
  arthritis and, 10
  esophageal cancer and, 21
  geriatric nutrition and, 55-56
  immunity and, 89-90
  lactation and, 135
  low-birth-weight and, 137
  non-insulin-dependent diabetes, 32
  pancreatic insufficiency and, 95
  peptic ulcers and, 47
  preconception nutrition and, 128
  pregnancy and, 130
  tissue healing and, 111